In *Whole Body Vibration*, B... siderable science behind vibrating for health. Testosterone and growth hormones increase and cortisol (stress hormone) decreases significantly! WBV helps reverse osteoporosis, increases leg strength, decreases fat in muscles, and improves bone density of spine and legs. It is equal to resistance training in improving leg strength and performance. *And, most of all, it is energizing!*

—C. Norman Shealy, MD, PhD
President, Holos Institutes of Health
Neurosurgeon, Author, and Worldwide Speaker

Whole Body Vibration is a compelling and entertaining look at the myriad and amazing benefits of WBV. I, myself, use my vibration plate every day because, simply put, *it just makes me feel good.*

—Frankie Boyer
Radio Personality
The Frankie Boyer Show

During more than twenty years of hosting *Strategies for Living Radio*, I've been privileged to talk to many innovators, and Becky Chambers is definitely one of them. Becky's work has been instrumental in changing the way we look at being "healthy" in the twenty-first century. Pioneers such as Becky are putting healthcare back where it belongs—in our own hands. Pardon the pun, but I get good vibrations from Becky Chambers and *Whole Body Vibration: The Future of Good Health*; I recommend you read it and consider its important message.

David McMillian, LPC-S, LMFT,
Marriage and Family Therapist

Becky presents state-of-the-art information on the exciting new technology of Whole Body Vibration in her book, *Whole Body Vibration: The Future of Good Health,* and I am happy to endorse it. I have been very impressed with Whole Body Vibration since I first learned about it when looking for treatment for a patient with severe osteoporosis who had no ability to exercise. WBV worked beautifully, resulting in a dramatic increase in bone density for my patient in just one year. The more I learn about WBV, the more impressed I am.

WBV can be used in both sickness and health. It can increase muscle strength and improve muscle tone and influence mood by improving neurotransmitter balance. It can have a positive impact on people with Metabolic Syndrome (increased blood pressure, high blood sugar levels, excess body fat around the waist, and lipid abnormalities). WBV is used by physical therapists, as well as professional athletes, to help heal injuries and improve conditioning. It even seems to have a positive impact on the endocrine system by increasing testosterone levels and decreasing cortisol levels (suggesting that it can reduce the impact of stress on us). I expect we will see much wider use of WBV in the future.

—John Bordiuk, MD
Internist and Medical Director
Inner Balance Integrative Medicine

I highly recommend whole body vibration for detoxification, lymphatic health, and bone health in my medical and surgical practice. Becky Chambers's book is a great source of information on this innovative health modality that even patients with significant health conditions find easy to incorporate into their routines.

—Susan E. Kolb, MD, FACS, ABIHM, Plastic Surgeon, Author of *The Naked Truth about Breast Implants*, and Host of the *Temple of Health Radio Show*

I had the pleasure of interviewing Becky Chambers on the *Nancy Ferrari Show* last year to talk about her book, *Whole Body Vibration: The Future of Good Health*, and I was very impressed with her knowledge and expertise on the technology and benefits of using WBV machines. Becky's passion about living a healthy life is truly what is needed by us all!

—Nancy Ferrari, CEO, Nancy Ferrari Media and Mentoring

More than ever, many of us are interested in living healthy, vibrant lives—especially as we age—and just like Becky, my life mission has become about feeling good, feeling strong, and incorporating healthy habits and practices into my everyday life. I am so grateful to Becky for sharing her knowledge about breakthrough body and mind energy therapies. It certainly gives me hope now and for the future.

—Ann Quasman, Chief Fulfillment Officer and Creator of *WomanTalk Live* and the *Conscious Conversations Café*

Whole Body Vibration
The Future of Good Health

Becky Chambers

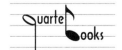

This book is written as a source of information to educate the readers. It is
not intended to replace medical advice or care, whether provided by a primary care physician, specialist, or other healthcare professional, including a
licensed alternative medical practitioner. Please consult your doctor before
beginning any form of health program. Neither the author nor the publisher
shall be liable or responsible for any adverse effects arising from the use or
application of any of the information contained herein, nor do they guaran-
tee that everyone will benefit or be healed by these techniques or practices,
nor are they responsible if individuals do not so benefit.

Cover design by Darryl Khalil
Cover art © ostill/Shutterstock.com and Eliks/Shutterstock.com
Photos in chapter 1 by Melinda Gordon
Author photo by Melinda Gordon
Interior design by Jane Hagaman

Quartet Books
Charlottesville, VA
www.quartetbooks.com

If you are unable to order this book from your local bookseller, you may order
directly from the author at her website: www.BCVibrantHealth.com.

Library of Congress Control Number: 2013903969

ISBN 978-0-9890662-0-4
10 9 8 7 6 5 4 3 2
Printed on acid-free paper in the United Sates

To Victor, my greatest challenge not including myself.

Challenges lead to growth;

so, in the end, my challenges have been gifts.

Author's Note

As of August 2014, rapid changes in the marketplace have prompted me to update chapter 8, Choosing a Vibration Machine. There are great new and very inexpensive options, as well as other innovations in vibration technology. In this revised chapter, I also address common confusing issues and misunderstandings.

Contents

Preface

I am a classic "canary in the mine." Forty years ago, my body began rebelling against the stresses of modern life by developing a host of chronic health issues. Those issues started when I was a young child with depression, which became chronic, at times severe, and continued for thirty years; along with this, I had crippling insecurities and self-esteem issues. I developed addictive and emotional eating behaviors, including bulimia, and by my early twenties, I weighed two hundred pounds. By then, I also had rampant allergies, painful digestive problems, immune system weakness, and numerous disabling joint and nervous system problems. Back then, I was an isolated freak of nature; today my experiences are becoming commonplace, as chronic health issues are skyrocketing. Forty years ago, I began my search for health and happiness. Listen to my hard-earned knowledge and experience now, and you may save yourself time, money, pain, and misery. You may even find joy, love, and success.

I began my search in my teens, using Western medicine and psychiatric care. For years there was little progress, and by my early twenties, the physical complaints urgently demanded attention. Out of desperation I began considering natural health, but by then so many systems in my body were involved and the situation was so complex that I was a difficult case.

For example, I had a terrible case of *Candida* (yeast) overgrowth. This is a gut flora disorder that in severe cases can become systemic, causing multiple symptoms and great distress. I would improve with diet changes and products or drugs to control the yeast, but within weeks I would be sick again because I had become allergic to whatever product I was taking. Because of this extreme reactivity, I was called a "universal reactor" and eventually ended up allergic to more than three hundred different foods. For many years, I was only able to eat by taking daily allergy desensitization drops and rotating all foods so that no food was repeated within a five-day period.

I tried many different natural-health approaches and doctors: special diets, nutritional supplements, herbs, Chinese medicine, chiropractic care, acupuncture, homeopathy, heavy-metal removal by intravenous and oral chelation, allergy desensitization, and more, but I was still going downhill. By my thirties, I could barely eat anything and had lost eighty pounds, ending up a slim 120 pounds of unhealthy, depressed, and lonely misery. My immune system was so overworked and weak that the slightest nick in my skin would inevitably lead to an infection that would take months to heal. My liver was so overwhelmed that I had developed multiple chemical sensitivity (MCS); I could eat only organic food and could not tolerate drugs of any sort. I figured I would eventually get some sort of serious infection, and because antibiotics only made me worse, I would probably die.

A key turning point came when I discovered Whole Body Vibration (WBV) about ten years ago and experienced its vast potential to improve health. Using WBV in combination with nutrition, supplements, and homeopathy, under the guidance of the talented Keith DeOrio, MD, I finally began to truly heal. Eventually, I began using WBV in my own natural healthcare consulting practice, becoming the first person in the northeast to use and supply WBV to the public. Without a doubt, WBV does have enormous potential to help people, but like any very powerful instrument, if it is used improperly, it can cause problems. I have written this book to help people take advantage of the many benefits of WBV without stumbling into the pitfalls. As a naturopath (natural health practitioner), I have seen that WBV works best with an understanding of the basic natural-health concepts of nutrition, the impact of toxins on our bodies, and chi energy—or our life force.

Acknowledgments

I want to thank all the many people who have helped me to learn and write about Whole Body Vibration (WBV). First, I want to thank my clients, who, over the last ten years, have helped me to learn how best to use WBV to help people. I'd particularly like to thank those clients who have generously allowed the use of their experiences and names to personalize and enliven this book: Frankie Boyer, Monica Calzolari, Doreen Hadge, Richard Hawkins, Ellen Lehn, Ann L. MacGibbon, Wendy MacLean, Mary Onorato, Hillary Repucci, Robert Williams, and Wayne Young.

For the excellent photos of WBV in action, I thank Linda Tighe, a client and the model, and Melinda Gordon, the photographer.

A heartfelt thanks also to my family and friends, who have provided support and encouragement throughout the years. Special thanks and love to my mother, Claire Smith, who provided editorial skills and financial backing.

I thank Dr. Keith DeOrio for many years of excellent medical care that helped me to achieve the higher level of physical and mental health that has made my work and writing possible. I thank Jeanne Mayell for her continuing wise advice regarding my life and for her help in the development of this book, including the idea to write the book in the first place.

I thank the following people for their essential and excellent professional services: editor, Tania Seymour; interior book designer, Jane Hagaman; cover designer, Darryl Khalil; and publicist, Sara Sgarlat.

Introduction

Whole Body Vibration (WBV) is exploding in popularity around the world because of its remarkable capacity to enhance health and well-being. WBV has been shown by extensive research over forty years to be intensive exercise, and movement is what we are designed for—it is the true fountain of youth but is often missing from our busy and sedentary modern lifestyles. As hard as it is to believe without actually experiencing it, ten minutes of WBV training will give you the benefits of one hour of conventional weight lifting, including increased muscle strength, bone density, flexibility, coordination, balance, and weight

Ten minutes of WBV training will give you the benefits of one hour of conventional weight lifting, including increased muscle strength, bone density, flexibility, coordination, balance, and weight loss.

loss. These benefits alone are enough to drive WBV's great popularity, but, in fact, they are only the tip of the iceberg when it comes to the total effect on health and well-being.

> WBV machines were initially invented for the Russian space program in the 1970s to counteract the effects of zero gravity and as a training method for their Olympic athletes. In the 1990s, after the fall of the Iron Curtain, commercial machines were developed and rapidly spread throughout Europe. Ten years later, vibration machines arrived in California and began to be available across the United States. Currently WBV is predominately known and used for its dramatic effects on the musculoskeletal system, and there are many companies making vibration machines.

When you stand on a vibration plate, you can feel the vibrations going through your body with a sensation similar to a massage. It seems so simple, but every cell and molecule in your body vibrates, leading to a cascade of effects so astounding that I am regularly met with, "It's too good to be true!" It is true, though, and has been documented extensively by forty years of research. There are also millions of satisfied users worldwide, including top athletes such as Shaquille O'Neal and Trace Armstrong, sports franchises such as the Denver Broncos and Miami Dolphins, and celebrities such as Madonna, Clint Eastwood, and Tony Robbins.

Chapter 1 focuses on the effects of vibration on your muscles—involuntarily, all of your muscle fibers will be activated, tightening and relaxing at the same speed the plate is vibrating—twenty to fifty times per second. That effect, plus the increase in gravity as your muscles hold your weight against the vibration, leads to the revolutionary result: ten minutes of WBV equals one hour of conventional weight lifting.

In chapter 2, I look at one of the most hotly pursued goals of modern life: losing weight! Just like exercise, WBV increases your metabolism and muscle strength, both of which help you burn more calories and lose weight. Just as important, WBV raises serotonin levels; this has powerful antidepressant effects and improves mood and sleep. Since many people overeat for emotional reasons rather than physical hunger, this effect can be a critical element in the battle to maintain and/or achieve a healthy weight.

Chapter 3 addresses the issue of bone-density loss and WBV's capacity to stimulate bone growth. WBV was, in fact, originally developed forty years ago in Russia to counteract the devastating effects of zero gravity on their cosmonauts in outer space. It turns out that vibration transmitted to the bones through muscle is exactly the signal your body needs to increase bone density. For millions in this country and worldwide who are facing the dangers of weakened bones and the lack of safe and effective treatment, this is exciting news indeed.

Another life-changing aspect of WBV is described in chapter 4: its effects on the nervous system and brain. WBV rapidly raises the levels of two neurotransmitters, serotonin and norepinephrine, that have positive effects on mood and energy levels. In addition, exercise has been shown to be the most important factor for brain health, powerfully stimulating neural cell growth and strength. This is a godsend for everybody—certainly people facing neurological disease and disability but for all of us really. Who couldn't use a little more brain power?

Feeling a lack of energy and zest? WBV may be just what you need. Chapter 5 looks at the numerous physiological effects of WBV that increase energy, including rising levels of testosterone (linked to both men's and women's sexual libidos and energy levels). WBV also increases circulation, bringing nutrients and oxygen to all cells, and the antidepressant effect also sends new energy through your mind and body. In addition, WBV works in ways similar to acupuncture to stimulate your electromagnetic energy, now acknowledged by Western medicine as well as Eastern traditions as the basis of our neurological system and thus connected to all parts of our bodies. For example, like acupuncture, WBV often rapidly lowers pain and inflammation levels.

Chapter 6 focuses on three common casualties of aging: sex, beauty, and mobility. The rejuvenating effects of WBV in all of these areas can be attributed in part to increasing human growth hormone, the body's major repair, regrowth, and anti-aging hormone. This effect of WBV, plus the increases in testosterone, circulation, and electromagnetic energy, combine to give you a whole new lease on life.

In chapter 7, I address the role of toxins in health and how WBV helps your body to eliminate toxins. In fact, because WBV has such a powerful detoxification effect, it is usually the limiting factor for most people using WBV. I suggest caution; start slow, with just a minute or two, and increase slowly. In this case, truly, less is more—but can you imagine an exercise system where the biggest problem is not to do too much?!

In chapter 8, we will take a look at the plethora of WBV machines now available: what the parameters of the different machines are, what to look for, and what to avoid. Which machine is best for you?

WBV is a powerful tool in the search for health and happiness, with an unprecedented ability to work on physical, mental, and energetic levels all at once. In a ten-minute session, you can essentially get the benefits of a workout, a massage, acupuncture, and a powerful detoxification treatment and achieve life-changing benefits for many aspects of physical and mental health.

chapter 1

The Ten-Minute Workout

The Revolution of Whole Body Vibration (WBV)

We all know we should be exercising, right? The problem lies in actually doing it. There has been a hilarious ad on TV recently about a couple who has joined a health club, but they never go. Every day they have a new excuse: too busy, had to work late, too tired, forgot my sneakers, lost my hair band, my mother called! It gets more and more ridiculous, but we're laughing in sympathy because we've all been there.

But what if exercising was so quick, enjoyable, relaxing, and conveniently located in your own home (or nearby) that it was the highlight of your day? If every day you could hardly wait to get to it, and you had to restrain yourself from doing too much? It is possible. Whole Body Vibration has arrived and just in time! We are a nation and world in desperate need of the many life-changing benefits of WBV.

Exercise: The Fountain of Youth

Our bodies are designed for physical activity, and they thrive on it. For example, exercise increases your circulation, bringing essential nutrients and oxygen to every part of your body, including your brain, and removing waste products. Amping up this process helps every cell and organ in your body to function at a higher level. And just by exercising, you increase your body's ability to drive the circulatory system. Your heart, which pumps your blood through the arteries on its outgoing journey, becomes stronger. Exercising builds more muscle, which in turn massages the veins in the gentler but essential pumping action that moves the blood on its return trip to the heart. Exercise, whether in a more traditional form or now with WBV, is also critical to maintaining muscle tone, bone density, and a healthy weight.

Our bodies are designed for physical activity, and they thrive on it.

Exercise and Your Brain

Just as important, exercise helps your mood and brain. If you are so depressed and lethargic that you can barely get out of your chair and exercise, sometimes your whole life can seem like an insurmountable mountain. The good news is that the very act of exercising will increase the levels of natural chemicals in your brain called neurotransmitters; this will raise your spirits, energize you, and help your brain to function better. Plus, exercise has actually been shown to increase the number of neurons and neural connections in your brain. These are important components of intelligence, so you will actually be getting smarter as you exercise.

The Ten-Minute WBV Workout

Now that you're raring to go and ready to start your new life as a fit, slim, and brilliant citizen of the world, what should you do first? WBV is a fantastic place to start, or use it as an addition to any fitness program already in place. Why? It is a quick, highly adaptable workout that can be tailored to any level of fitness: from the couch potato to the occasional jogger, the tennis player to the weekend warrior, the amateur athlete all the way up to the elite professional athlete. At the easiest beginner level, and on extra-lazy days, you simply stand on the gently vibrating plate, receiving a vibration that will feel like a massage. Through the involuntary automatic activation of your nervous system, and thus your muscles, you will still be experiencing a mild workout. At the other end of the spectrum: Ten minutes of WBV equals one hour of conventional weight lifting.

Ten minutes of WBV equals one hour of conventional weight lifting.

At first that may seem impossible, just too good to be true—but it is true. While the exact ratio does depend on which machine you use and how you use it (whether you work out or just stand on the plate), forty years of research and the devotion of thousands of professional athletes and elite users, including Shaquille O'Neil, Jane Fonda, Madonna, the Denver Broncos, and the Tennessee Titans, attest to WBV's effectiveness.

How Whole Body Vibration Creates Intensive Exercise

♦ Holding weight against vibration increases the effects of gravity. Because of this physical reality (described mathematically as gravity equals mass times acceleration), when vibrating, your muscles must hold up to three times your actual weight, the exact amount depending on the amplitude and frequency of the vibration. If you have any doubt about this, consider the arm and shoulder muscle development of men who operate jackhammers.

♦ Every muscle fiber will automatically tense and relax at the same rate that the machine is vibrating, usually twenty to fifty times per second. That adds up to one thousand to three thousand little tiny "reps" per minute—much more work for your muscles than holding a position (isometric exercise) or typical repetition workouts.

♦ One hundred percent of your muscles will be working, while in traditional exercises, only some of your muscles are engaged. For example, in a nonvibrating squat, only about 40 percent of your leg muscles are working, but if you are vibrating, 100 percent of your leg muscles will be firing.

The combination of these three factors results in an intensive workout, in which, by the end of one minute, your muscles may be begging for relief. If it is still not hard enough, one can also carry weights, which will rapidly increase the effort as the gravitational increase from the vibration will double or triple any weight increase.

You can also vary the type of exercise position to change which muscle groups must work to hold your weight. For example, you can do push-ups for upper-body strength, or sit on the plate in a V shape (see page 10) to work the abdominal muscles. There are endless variations of positions to engage different muscle groups. A typical workout includes one-minute intervals in numerous different positions to achieve the effect of a full-body workout in ten minutes.

While circulation does increase with WBV, this is partly due to the massaging action of

Holding weight against vibration increases the effects of gravity. . . . Every muscle fiber will automatically tense and relax at the same rate that the machine is vibrating, usually twenty to fifty times per second. . . . One hundred percent of your muscle will be working, while in traditional exercises, only some of your muscles are engaged.

the muscle fibers as they tense and relax. WBV does not provide intensive aerobic exercise, so you should also incorporate some type of aerobic exercise into your total fitness plan, such as walking, biking, running, swimming, etc. You will probably find it much easier to do this when you are using WBV because of the powerful energizing and mood-elevating effects.

Six Sample Exercise Positions, Massages, and Stretches

There are as many positions possible on the vibration plate as you can think of. Anything is fine; experiment and see what feels good. Even if you just stand on the vibrating plate, you will be getting enormous benefits, though the muscle-strengthening effect is greatest when holding exercise positions. Here are a few standard positions designed to target major muscle groups for strengthening, massaging, or stretching. For pictures of many more suggested exercise positions, check the WBV pages of my website at www.BCVibrantHealth.com. Or you can buy a chart with thirty suggested WBV positions at Amazon.com. Search for "Beginner's Whole Body Vibration Exercise Chart." For isometric exercises, you get into a position and hold it. For more intensive kinetic exercises, you can move slowly in and out of the position.

Caution: *Because of the powerful detoxification effects of Whole Body Vibration (see chapter 7), you must start slowly, often doing no more than one minute per day, then build up your time slowly.*

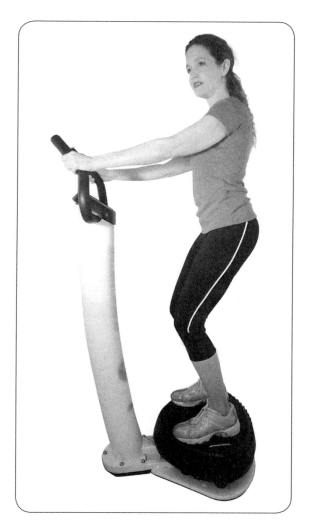

1. **Beginner's Position:** Stand in a comfortable, balanced position with knees slightly flexed. If you enjoy the sensation of the vibration (and you have no back or neck problems), you can straighten your legs and more vibration will travel up through your bones to your entire body. Personally, I love this sensation, but if you don't like the vibration in your head, keep your knees bent.

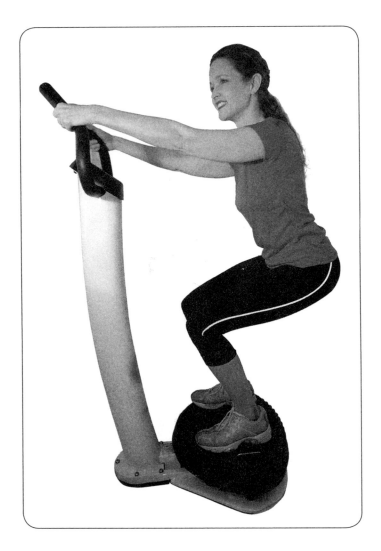

2. Deep Squat: Position your feet in the middle of the plate, slightly apart. Bend your knees about eighty degrees. Don't let your knees extend beyond your toes. Arch your back, keep your head up, and maintain balance. This position feels sort of like going to sit in a chair, then holding that position. This exercise targets leg muscles.

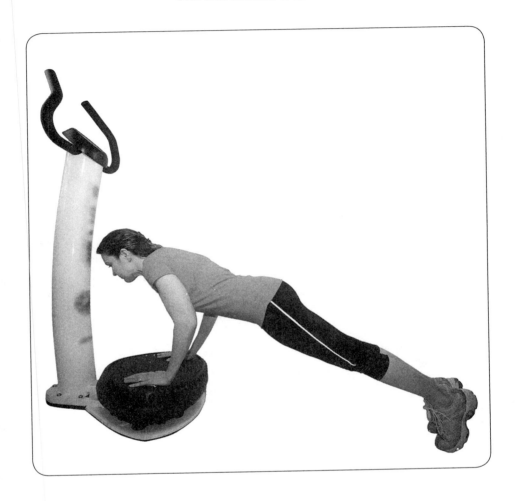

3. **Push-Up:** Facing the plate, put your hands flat on the outer edges and keep your feet on the ground behind the plate. Keep your back straight, shoulders over your hands, and stomach in. If this is too hard, you can rest your knees on the ground. This position targets chest, arms, and back muscles.

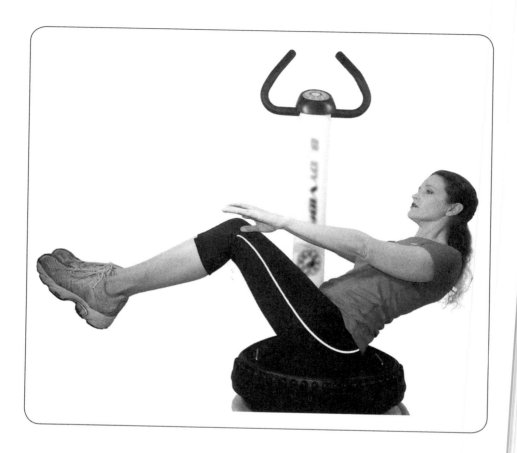

4. **Basic Abdominal:** Sit sideways on the plate on a small mat or towel, assuming a V-shaped position, leaning back and lifting legs. The straighter the legs in this position, the harder it will be. Try with bent knees first. This exercise targets abdominal muscles, which are essential for good posture and help prevent lower back pain.

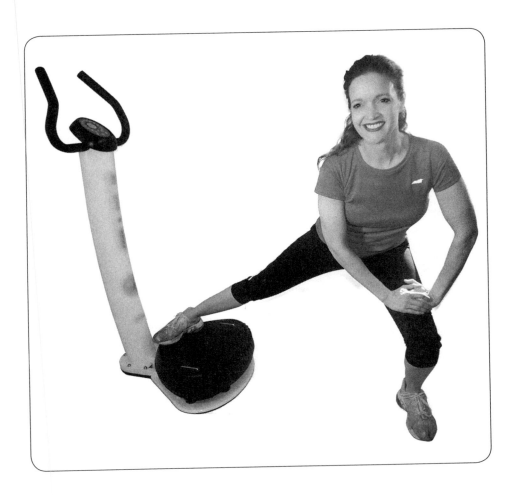

5. **Adductor Stretch:** Stand in front of the plate, facing sideways. Place one foot on the plate, toward the back of the
   plate, so that your leg is stretched. With your weight on
   the leg on the floor, bend that knee and rest both hands
   on that knee. Slowly tense the inner thigh of the leg on
   the plate.

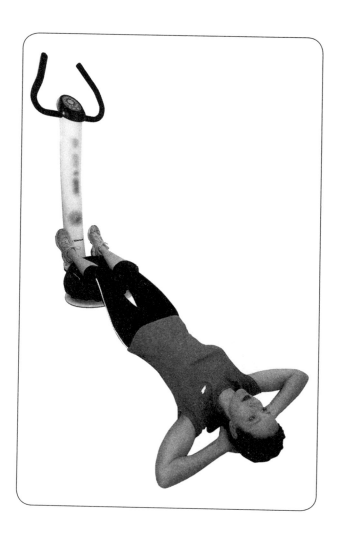

6. **Calves Massage:** Place your calves on the plate, lie back on floor behind you, hands behind your head, and relax. This is super relaxing and a favorite position for many people.

chapter 2

Losing Weight with Whole Body Vibration

Why Vibration?

Whole Body Vibration helps you lose weight by speeding up your metabolism, increasing energy levels, elevating your mood, and strengthening muscles, even if all you do is stand on the vibrating plate. Now you might be laughing and making a joke about those vibrating belts from the 1960s, but don't let the laughter stop you! Scientific research has shown increased weight and fat loss with WBV, along with many other benefits, and my own extensive experience with clients and myself makes it clear that WBV is a huge plus in any weight-loss program.

Weight loss is a national obsession, and there are good reasons for this. It is clear that weight gain and obesity are major health risks and have a long list of associated diseases. In modern times, with our sedentary lifestyles and easy access to unhealthy but addictive and high-calorie foods, weight gain has become a huge problem. However, the psychological toll of this societal problem can be devastating, and I urge keeping things in perspective. Fat, a natural element of our bodies that in small amounts is important to good health, historically has been essential to our survival as a species and makes for lovely soft and smooth contours. And if you've got too much, you can always lose some!

I had a marvelous conversation with an African woman a few years ago. I was complaining about a couple of pounds I had gained, and she told me that she was trying to *gain* weight, that she thought she looked unattractive and unhealthy at only 165 pounds. Then she told me that in *her* country, I would have to spend at least a month or two in the "fattening hut," or no man would want me, and I would never marry. What a breath of fresh air!

What we actually see as beautiful and attractive is blooming vibrant health, because that means you'll clearly be around for a long time, creating a wonderful life and helping all your loved ones to live similarly long and happy lives. The great gift of WBV is that it will help you not only to lose weight, but it will improve your physical and mental health in many other ways at the same time.

How Whole Body Vibration Helps You Lose Weight

- ♦ WBV can be an intense workout, and, like any workout, this will increase your metabolic rate so that you burn more calories and lose weight more easily—and the time required to achieve the same results as with traditional exercise forms is much less. Remember: ten minutes of WBV equals one hour of conventional weight training.

- ♦ The workout will build lean muscle mass that will continue to burn more calories all day long. Lean muscle mass can account for 60 percent of your energy and calorie expenditure while at rest.

- ♦ WBV raises serotonin levels in your brain, which has a powerful antidepressant effect (see also chapter 4). With your mental state happier and calmer, it will be easier for you to eat properly and exercise. Everybody knows they should eat well (probably lesser quantities as well as healthier choices) and exercise more to lose weight; the problem is actually doing it. WBV helps you to be in that calm and relaxed but energized mental state in which you can focus and achieve your goals.

- ♦ WBV gives you strength (increased muscle power) and energy (see also chapter 5). So when you do go out to exercise—now more often because you have more energy and you are in a better emotional and mental state—you will work harder, consequently burning more calories.

- ♦ WBV lowers cortisol levels.[1] Cortisol is a major stress and aging hormone that promotes fat production and storage. Lowering cortisol levels helps promote fat burning and proper fat metabolism.

- ♦ WBV improves joint health in numerous ways (see chapter 6) so that you have greater mobility and are able to exercise more.

Here's a frequently asked question: Will people see my fat jiggle?

No, don't worry! Only your feet will visibly vibrate.

Scientific Research

A 2010 study of sixty-one overweight and obese adults saw significant weight loss with a combination of WBV and diet, and the best long-term results were obtained for those participants combining WBV with aerobic exercise and diet. Their conclusions were that

> combining either aerobic exercise or WBV training with caloric restrictions can help to achieve a sustained long-term weight loss of 5–10%. . . . WBV training may have the potential to reduce VAT [visceral adipose tissue; i.e., fat] more than aerobic exercise in obese adults. . . . Only Fitness and Vibration (participants) managed to maintain a weight loss of 5% or more in the long term.[2]

In a study in 2007 of mice that received fifteen minutes of daily vibration, the mice that got vibration ended up with 27 percent lower amounts of fat, along with corresponding increases in bone density, than the control mice that didn't get any vibration.[3] In the photo from this study, the dark areas are fat, and the mice who received vibration are visibly considerably leaner and have less of the dark fat areas.

MICE EXPOSED TO VIBRATION   **NORMAL MICE**

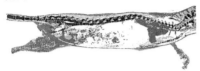   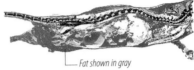

Fat shown in gray

Source: Clinton Rubin; PANS. Used by permission of Dr. Clinton Rubin.

Preliminary (unpublished) research conducted at the Sana-derm Health Clinic in Germany on the effects of vibration-enhanced exercise training for cellulite reduction and fat loss demonstrated that six months of training a maximum of eleven minutes on the vibration platform reduced cellulite by 25.68 percent. In addition, when vibration was combined with aerobic activity for forty minutes, the study participants experienced a 32 percent reduction in cellulite.

Another unpublished preliminary trial evaluated the effect of vibration training in comparison to traditional training methods over a period of six weeks. Body fat was reduced by 11.2 percent with vibration as compared to 10.6 percent in the traditional training group. Body-fat reduction was greater in the vibration group, and the total exercise time was considerably less. (Pneumex Equipment and S. Sordorff, PT; Sandpoint, Idaho)

Combining either aerobic exercise or WBV training with caloric restrictions can help to achieve a sustained long-term weight loss of 5–10%. . . . WBV training may have the potential to reduce VAT more than aerobic exercise. . . .

Another preliminary (and unpublished) study evaluated the effects of vibration training on weight loss. In this study, the vibration-training group had a net increase of 12 percent in their resting metabolic rate after three months. Consequently, WBV can allow one to burn more calories compared to inactive individuals. (Slim & Shape Centers Inc., Windsor, Canada)

Troubleshooting

While I have seen excellent results with many clients (and myself: I once weighed two hundred pounds but have now been 125 pounds for many years), there can be other issues that need to be addressed. If you are not losing weight and inches while using WBV, aerobically exercising, and eating a healthy diet, possible reasons include:

1. **Too much vibration too soon:** This is the most common mistake. Vibration is a very powerful detoxification system (see chapter 7), so many people will need to start at just one minute on a gentle machine and slowly build up the time and vibration frequency. Too much vibration too soon can stress your body, leading to temporary detoxification overload so that you do not see the beneficial effects. Though it is hard to believe, the first thing to try if you are not seeing weight loss is to vibrate less. Everybody wants to vibrate more, thinking more exercise will help. But in this case, because the detoxification effect is so great, *less is more*. I see the best results with my clients when we start with one minute and increase slowly.

2. **Candida yeast:** Candida yeast overgrowth is an epidemic in this country and can cause gas, bloating, and water retention, as well as sugar and carbohydrate cravings and many other symptoms. (See resources and additional reading for further information.) Used properly, WBV will help to eliminate yeast because WBV is such a powerful health-enhancing system. The more you strengthen your overall health, which is linked to your immune system, the less yeast will be able to survive. But because WBV is also a powerful detoxification system, too much WBV can temporarily weaken your immune system, leading to yeast levels increasing, along with the associated symptoms.

Everybody wants to vibrate more, thinking more exercise will help. But in this case, because the detoxification effect is so great, less is more.

So, again, it is important to start with just a small amount of WBV, sometimes just thirty seconds to one minute a day, and to increase slowly. Exactly how much WBV a person will be able to tolerate without aggravating their symptoms varies greatly depending on their overall state of health and the amount of toxicity in their tissues. Thus it's useful to work with a qualified professional.

3. **Hormonal and metabolic imbalances:** If you have eliminated the first two, and most likely, causes for not losing weight, you are left with hormonal and metabolic imbalances. There are numerous hormonal and metabolic issues that can make it difficult to lose weight. Consult the additional reading list and/or a qualified health professional to address these issues and continue with your WBV program.

chapter 3

Increasing Bone Density

Building Bone Safely and Naturally

WBV is famous for promoting bone growth. Extensive research over the last forty years has shown that WBV safely promotes and increases bone density, more so than conventional exercise, which has long been understood to be important for healthy bone development. This breakthrough is of critical importance to space travelers, who lose bone density at a rate of up to one hundred times faster than a normal person on earth,[1] and to postmenopausal women in developed countries, who are experiencing epidemic levels of bone loss. Add to this scenario the very real dangers associated with bone-density drugs, and you have a lifesaving technology that has spurred hundreds of studies and interest all over the world.

Research results with animals and younger, healthy people have been dramatic. The development and use of vibration in the 1970s allowed Russian cosmonauts to be in space twice as long as their nonvibrating American counterparts (approximately two hundred days versus one hundred days). More recently, a NASA website cited the effects of vibration on turkeys, sheep, and rats as "profound . . . promoting near-normal rates of bone formation"[2] under laboratory conditions simulating the zero gravity conditions of space flight. In other research, Dr. Clinton Rubin, director of the Center for Biotechnology at the State University of New York at Stony Brook, reported increasing the bone density in mice nearly 30 percent with vibration for fifteen minutes a day for fifteen weeks.[3] And a research study with a well-trained cyclist showed an increase in bone density of 1.6 percent in just ten weeks.[4]

The results with postmenopausal women show not only increases in bone density, but also improvements in other critical areas affecting the risk of falls. One recent six-month study of ninety women concluded that

> **strength increased as much as 16 percent in upper leg muscles, while bone density at the hip increased by 1.5 percent. In addition, the whole body vibration group showed an improvement in postural control and balance, increased muscle strength, and lean mass while losing body fat and fat mass.[5]**

While this study is encouraging, there are other studies concluding that vibration did not increase bone density in postmenopausal women.[6] The studies with animals and younger people demonstrate clearly that WBV does stimulate bone to increase its density, but building bone is a complex process involving the healthy functioning of many different systems. As people age, many systems in their bodies do not work as well, so just providing the signal to build bone may not be a sufficient intervention by itself.

A critical missing element in the studies with older people is comprehensive nutritional supplementation. Studies on bone density typically provide participants with, at most, calcium, magnesium, and vitamin D, but bone building is a complex process requiring more than a dozen critical nutrients, and older people often have decreased nutrient intake and absorption.

My clients, who receive more extensive supplementation along with WBV, see impressive results. For example, Mary Onorato, a seventy-year-old woman whose doctor told her that going over a bump in the road or coughing too hard could cause a fracture in her vertebrae because her bone-density test put her in the category of "extremely severe" bone-density loss, experienced a complete reversal of bone loss in two and a half years to where she now has the "bones of a healthy young woman" (see page 30 for more details on Mary's remarkable reversal of osteoporosis).

How WBV Increases Bone Density

Research by Dr. Rubin, through his work with Marodyne Medical and the LivMD low-intensity vibration device, has shown that it is small, high-frequency signals that cause bone

to grow, a sort of buzz or vibration received from muscle attach-
ments to bone,[7] not high-impact signals as was once thought. In
other words, it is not the impact of a person's foot against the
ground that signals bone to grow, but rather the quivering of
muscle fibers against bone as the muscle fibers contract in the
process of running.

WBV provides this same type of small high-frequency signals to many areas and bones intensively, all at once, and with
minimal effort. Just standing on a vibrating plate will cause
all muscle fibers connected to weight-bearing bone to
involuntarily contract and release twenty to fifty times
per second. To impact the arms, hands, wrists, and shoulders, different positions would be recommended, such as a
push-up, to activate muscles attached to these bones.

WBV provides . . . small high-frequency signals to many areas and bones intensively, all at once, and with minimal effort. Just standing on a vibrating plate will cause all muscle fibers . . . to involuntarily contract and release twenty to fifty times per second.

The power and size of the vibration machine also affects
muscle activation, with a greater amplitude vibration transmitting the signal to more
of the body, but larger more powerful machines are also more
expensive and have more powerful detoxification effects, so
they are not always the best choice for an individual (see also
chapters 7 and 8). Most of the bone-density research has been

done on relatively gentle low-power machines (1–2 mm amplitude with a gravitational force of less than 1.25), so as long as enough time is spent on these machines in varying positions (ten to twenty minutes per day), they should be sufficient.

Double Motor Vibration Machines

To achieve greater power, thus a greater workout effect, many WBV machines have two motors in them. However, it is impossible to ever completely synchronize two motors. This results in a desynchronizing message sent to your nervous system and energy field, which can have negative consequences over time (see chapter 8).

Bone-Density Drugs

Poor nutrition, a lack of exercise, and the use of numerous drugs that inhibit proper digestion and assimilations of nutrients and/or bone development have combined to create an epidemic of weak and brittle bones. Statistically, in the US, one third of women and one sixth of men will now experience a hip-bone fracture at some point in their lifetime, and these types of fractures often result in death or permanent loss of independence and mobility.[8]

In response, the pharmaceutical industry and Western medicine have developed, and heavily promoted, a class of drugs called bisphosphonates. These include all those drugs advertised by poorly informed movie stars and celebrities on TV: Fosamax, Actonel, Boniva, and Reclast. These drugs do result in bone-density tests showing an increase in bone density—but beware! These drugs achieve an increase in bone density by halting your body's natural ability to reabsorb old and damaged bone. The result is more bone, but it is weak, old, and fragile bone.

The situation is most acute in the jawbone, where increased blood flow supports the extra bone repair that is normal in that area. This causes a concentration of the drugs and their effects and has led to a surge in cases of a horrifying condition called osteonecrosis (bone death) of the jaw (ONJ). Unfortunately, this process of bone death and rot is usually painless and hidden, so it goes unnoticed for years, until the person goes to the dentist for a surgical procedure. Then, with exposure to the bacteria in the mouth and the increased demand for healing, a major disaster follows, with permanent, untreatable pain; disfigurement; and great difficulty eating.[9]

Fosamax, Actonel, Boniva, and Reclast achieve an increase in bone density by halting your body's natural ability to reabsorb old and damaged bone.

Another area in which this drug-induced bone weakness is showing up is in a bizarre type of severe thigh-bone fracture that happens without any unusual stress on the bone. People who have been taking bisphosphonates for five or more years (though occasionally this problem shows up within months) are ending up in emergency rooms with cross-transverse compound fractures of the femur bone from merely standing up or walking.[10] These are still very rare occurrences, but they may be about to become more common as hundreds of thousands of Americans who have been on these drugs for many years reach the critical time period.

Normal Bone Growth

Healthy bone formation and growth is a complex process involving numerous systems in the body, including bone building and remodeling cells within the bone itself, digestion, hormones, the liver and kidneys, and the presence in plentiful amounts of more than a dozen minerals and vitamins. An excellent book in which this process is extensively researched and clearly detailed is *Your Bones: How You Can Prevent Osteoporosis and Have Strong Bones for Life—Naturally*, by Lara Pizzorno, the editor and author of numerous natural health publications and books.

Excellent nutrition and a healthy digestive system that is able to extract and absorb all the necessary nutrients are of critical importance to building bone. In addition to calcium, magnesium, and phosphorus, it is also necessary to have available the minerals strontium, boron, zinc, manganese, copper, silicon, molybdenum, and selenium and vitamins A, C, D, K1, K2, B6, B12, folate, and riboflavin.[11]

Luckily, a healthy diet for building bone is the same diet that is healthy for every other part of you. A primarily plant-based, whole-foods diet with small amounts of animal products if desired will make an enormous difference to your health. All parts and systems in your body will work better, and the nutrients that every part of your body requires to function are supplied. In deep and scary contrast is the average American diet with its heavy load of junk and fast food and mind-bogglingly tiny amounts of fruits and vegetables. The second National Health and Nutrition Examination Survey found that only 27 percent of Americans are eating three servings of fruits and vegetables per day, but this included potatoes, most of which were eaten as french fries and chips![12] Chips and fries don't count.

Within our bones, one type of specialized bone cell, called an osteoclast, breaks down old and worn-out bone. Another type of bone cell, called an osteoblast, is a bone-forming cell that pulls calcium, magnesium, and phosphorus from the blood to build new bone. Without the osteoclasts, damaged bone builds up, leading to weak bone; without healthy osteoblast activity, new bone will not be formed. Bisphosphonate drugs increase total bone density by killing the osteoclast cells; the result is weak and diseased bone. WBV will signal your body to increase bone density without interfering with the removal of old and weak bone.

Older People and Bone Growth

As people age, critical systems for bone building may not function as well; digestion and assimilation of nutrients may be poor; hormonal changes decrease bone building (especially in women); and older people are often taking drugs that interfere in some way with the process of building bone. For example, people with low stomach acid do not digest and absorb many nutrients (including only about 4 percent of the most commonly used form of calcium supplement, calcium carbonate), and studies have shown that about 40 percent of postmenopausal women are severely deficient in stomach acid.[13]

Even worse, many of these people will end up further compounding the problem by taking antacids (over-the-counter or prescription) for "acid reflux," when in fact the problem is poor digestion due to too little acid, not enough enzymes, or *Candida* yeast overgrowth, all of which could be resolved easily and quickly with natural treatments.[14]

Western medicine is notoriously poor in its understanding and approach to nutrition. So WBV bone-density studies do not provide the full range of necessary nutrients to participants. But you cannot build a house with only lumber and nails. You also need nail guns, workers, screws, measuring tools, siding, sheetrock, windows, doors, etc. It is the same with building bone— there are many critical elements, and nothing at all can happen without them. The vibration supplies the signal, something like a foreman yelling, "Let's go," and the calcium and magnesium could be the lumber, but where are the workers, nails, nail guns, etc.? What you end up with is a lot of lumber lying on the ground and a foreman yelling, "Let's go! Let's go!"

Nutritional Supplements

Healthy, whole-food choices are important, but the truth is that even with excellent food choices, because our food supply is so compromised by poor soils, overuse of nitrogen fertilizers, early picking, and long shipping and storage times, not to mention food processing that destroys the remaining nutrients, it can be very difficult to get enough nutrition to reverse existing health issues. For this reason, I generally recommend taking high-quality nutritional supplements along with eating a healthy diet. An excellent comprehensive mineral and vitamin bone-building supplement, providing more than two dozen nutrients important for bone growth, is a product called Pro-Bono, made by Ortho Molecular Products.

Documented Case Study

Mary Onorato has the most dramatic and well-documented case among my clients. Over the course of five years, she had four DEXA bone density tests (the gold standard of bone density testing) to track her extremely severe osteoporosis, all at the same hospital and with the same equipment. After two years of slowly declining bone density, despite a strict routine of comprehensive mineral and vitamin supplementation and regular weightlifting and walking, she found me and began WBV. At that point, she saw a sudden and dramatic turnaround (see graph on the following page).

Mary never took any bone-building prescription drugs and had stopped the weightlifting and walking several months prior to beginning WBV, but she had always continued with her nutritional supplements. The only change in her program once she met me was the addition of WBV. WBV clearly provides a powerful signal to your body to build bone. And given the right stimulus and nutritional support, nearly everyone can build bone.

Mary Onorato's Lumbar Spine Bone Density

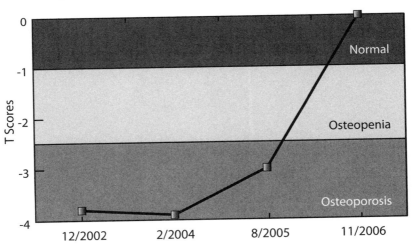

Note: Mary Onorato's results are not typical, but are so well documented and clear that I wanted to show her case. Most of my other postmenopausal clients with osteopenia or osteoporosis build bone at a slower rate, usually 2 to 6 percent over six months. These results are from my clients' bone-density studies as reported to me; they are not part of a published study. They are, however, significantly better than published studies of WBV's effect on bone building in postmenopausal women.

chapter 4

Get Smart and Protect Your Brain

A Wondrous Gift

Your brain, home of your mind and soul, connects you to everything in the universe and makes you a unique being of vast potential and ability. Through your mind and soul, you link to the knowledge of people from the past, present, and future; every aspect of the world around you; and your own body and existence. Through the nervous system and chi energy, the brain links to every organ, system, and molecule in the body. Thus a critical key to fulfilling your potential and finding a life of joy, love, and peace is to stimulate your brain to grow, reach its full potential, and stay healthy and vibrant well into old age.

The latest research is that nothing helps your brain develop and stay healthy more than exercise. A recent *New York Times* magazine article, "Jogging Your Brain," states, "For more than a decade, neuroscientists and physiologists have been gathering evidence of the beneficial relationship between exercise and brainpower. But the newest findings make it clear that this isn't just a relationship; it is *the* relationship. . . . Exercise, the latest neuroscience suggests, does more to bolster thinking than thinking does."[1]

Exercise, the latest neuroscience suggests, does more to bolster thinking than thinking does.

WBV has been proven beyond a doubt to be intensive exercise when used for that purpose. Hundreds of research studies, top athletes around the world, and, in fact, anybody who has ever tried working out on a powerful vibration plate with muscles begging for relief can attest to this. Yet, even if you only stand on a vibrating plate, you will be stimulating muscles to contract and neurons to fire twenty to fifty times per second, which adds up to ten to fifteen thousand times in one ten-minute session—massive neurological stimulation.

With a wide variety of possible positions on the plate and intensities of vibration, WBV can be adapted for all levels of physical ability. This allows almost anybody, from a pro athlete to a wheelchair-bound person, from a busy professional to a depressed, unmotivated low achiever, to experience the neurological and other benefits of exercise.

An Almost Inconceivably Complex Organ

Your brain contains one hundred to two hundred billion neurons (nerve cells). Each neuron connects to up to one thousand other neurons through dendrites (thin nerve-tissue filaments), which make up a branching treelike structure. These connections between neurons are called synapses, and there are some three hundred trillion synapses in a brain, creating vast networks of interconnected neurons. At each synapse, signals leap across a tiny "synaptic gap" via natural chemicals called neurotransmitters, activating an electrical signal that shoots through the next neuron. The latest research shows that there are one thousand activation sites for these neurotransmitters per synapse.

The result is a brain in which there are more neurons than people on earth, more synapses than stars in our galaxy, and more complexity than in all the computers on earth put together. Stretch out all those dendrites plus axons (the part of the neuron that is something like the trunk of a tree with a root system that connects to organs and tissues up to three feet away), and they would reach to the moon and back.

It is this very complexity, especially the number of connections between neurons, that gives us our intelligence. "Thinking" involves neurons sending electrochemical signals across the synaptic gaps, lighting up pathways throughout that vast network of billions of neurons in your brain.

Whole Body Vibration Is a Powerful Natural Antidepressant

Two neurotransmitters, serotonin and norepinephrine, have been shown to increase with WBV. Serotonin is a critical neurotransmitter in your brain that contributes to sounder sleep and feelings of mastery, pleasure, and relaxation. This is the same neurotransmitter that is targeted by prescription antidepressant drugs such as Prozac and Wellbutrin, as well as many illegal drugs such as marijuana, cocaine, and Ecstasy. While prescription drugs for depression can be valuable for helping to alleviate symptoms, they also have side effects, and they can lead to increasing tolerance and dependence on those drugs. Whole Body Vibration is a natural, safe, rapid, nonaddictive, and legal way to increase serotonin and norepinephrine.

Whole Body Vibration is a natural, safe, rapid, nonaddictive, and legal way to increase serotonin and norepinephrine.

Norepinephrine is both a neurotransmitter and a hormone, and low levels of this essential molecule have been linked to depression and low energy. Norepinephrine (along with epinephrine) underlies the fight-or-flight response, giving the body sudden energy in times of stress; it increases the heart rate, triggers the release of glucose from energy stores, increases blood flow to skeletal muscles and oxygen supply to the brain, and it can suppress nerve inflammation.

Studies with rats have shown rapid increases in serotonin levels with WBV,[2] but physical measurements of brain serotonin levels can only be done in animals (as brain tissue samples must be taken). Anecdotal evidence of increased serotonin and norepinephrine levels with WBV is strong. Hundreds of my clients, and thousands of users around the world, report rapid and dramatic improvements in mood, energy, and sleep within days of beginning vibration. They also report increased motivation, focus, and activity levels. This is an area of great potential and should be investigated more thoroughly.

Hundreds of my clients report rapid and dramatic improvements in mood, energy, and sleep.

Testimonials

"Since I started vibrating two months ago, I am so much calmer and happier than I was—and sleeping more soundly. My kids say, 'Mom, you're definitely less uptight and angry.'"

—Monica Calzolari,
director of enrollment communications,
University of Massachusetts Boston

"I have become addicted to my vibration plate, even if it's only for a few minutes a day. It's my feel-good therapy—a day without vibrating is like a day without sunshine! It just makes you feel so good."

—Frankie Boyer, radio personality

"I am happier and have more energy now than I ever did when I was on Prozac."

—Anonymous

"I'm like the Energizer Bunny, my hay fever is gone, my mood is better and more stable, I lost 30 pounds, and am much stronger than I have ever been."

—Doreen Hadge, housecleaner

Neurogenesis and Plasticity

Neurogenesis is the creation of new brain cells. This was once thought to only happen before birth, but it is now known that, at a slower pace, neurogenesis does continue throughout life. This neurogenesis allows for brain "plasticity," meaning that it can continue to grow and change throughout life, making new neural connections that allow you to not only learn new skills and knowledge but to increase your ability to learn, think creatively, and change.

An amazing example of neurogenesis and brain plasticity later in life is a new therapy that has been developed for stroke victims who have been paralyzed. Intensive physical therapy for many hours per day with the paralyzed limb, while the normal arm and hand are immobilized, results in the regeneration of brain matter and physical function for people who have suffered complete paralysis of one arm and hand for as long as seventeen years.

Exercise triggers neurogenesis by prompting the production of brain-derived neurotropic factor (BDNF), which strengthens cells and axons and the connections among neurons, as well as sparking the formation of new neurons. BDNF is thus a physical mediator for increasing the complexity and strength of the neural network in the brain that reflects intellectual potential.

Research showing this connection between exercise and the brain has primarily been done with aerobic exercise. However, similar neurological and muscular processes are involved with weightlifting-type exercises, to which WBV is most similar. Perhaps WBV, with its massive neurological stimulation, will eventually be found to stimulate BDNF and brain development even more effectively than other forms of exercise; scientific research in this area is eagerly awaited.

Neurological Diseases

Early, short-term studies in the mid-2000s with Parkinson's patients were encouraging, showing significant improvements in several Parkinson's disease parameters: strength, balance, and rigidity. However, the conclusion of a review of thirteen more recently published articles regarding neurological diseases (five on Parkinson's, two on cerebral palsy, three on multiple sclerosis, and three on strokes) saw increases in strength, but no improvement in other areas, from one session and little overall benefit from longer-term use.[3]

I would suggest that these studies were not designed with an understanding of the critical issues of detoxification and nutritional support and that this doomed the results from the start. To realize the potential benefits of WBV, especially in weakened populations of people who already have disease, you must take these issues into consideration (see chapters 7 and 8).

There was a wide variation in the study protocols, but, in general, the studies gave elderly people with disease much more vibration than I, as an experienced naturopath and successful practitioner of WBV, would give to that population. One study gave thirty sessions of fifteen minutes of vibration per session in just five consecutive days to elderly people with Parkinson's (average age of seventy-four years).[4] I would not give this population *any* vibration without also giving them appropriate nutritional products, and then they would start at perhaps thirty *seconds* a couple of times a week at the lowest vibration settings.

Even in younger people without severe health issues, I generally see the best results starting with one minute and slowly building up over a period of several weeks to perhaps five minutes, depending on the individual.

Exhibit A: Becky Chambers

I spent forty years telling people that I couldn't write, that I had terrible writer's block and was too depressed and repressed to write. This was true, for forty years. Writing was a nightmare for most of my life, to the extent that I dropped out of a high-school course because I had to write a term paper and couldn't. I majored in biology at college, because I liked the subject but also because you didn't have to write papers.

I have exercised for most of my life, sometimes extensively (as my health would allow), and it did not noticeably affect either the depression or the writing issue. But from the time I started vibrating daily six years ago, plus taking many high-potency homeopathics that release negative repressive energy, my writing began to change dramatically. I have since written two books, the first a memoir of this transformative period, *Beyond the Great Abyss*, and this book on WBV. There is also a sequel to *Beyond the Great Abyss* due out soon. Turns out, I'm a writing dynamo!

Could You Use Some Brain Stimulation?

Are you reaching your potential? Who even knows what their potential is? I believe it is usually much greater than we realize, but life, poor health, environmental factors, and our own nega-tive thinking gets in our way. In addition, beginning in their late twenties, most people will lose about 1 percent annually of the cells in the hippocampus, a key portion of the brain related to memory and certain types of learning. Plus, as the brain is connected to all parts of the body, almost all health issues will improve with a better-functioning brain, especially depression, anxiety, memory loss, low energy, and nervous-system diseases. Give yourself the gift of Whole Body Vibration, and your brain will repay you with opportunities you cannot yet even imagine.

chapter 5

Boost Your Energy

Energy and Your Life

Busy, busy, busy . . . so much to do and so little time. For many people, modern life has become a race in which time is a scarce and precious commodity. Others have been running so hard and are so stressed that they have become chronically fatigued and can barely move anymore. But what if you could boost your physical energy level, balance and focus your mind, and raise your spiritual energy all at the same time? What might that do for you, for your ability to accomplish your goals, find your true path, and enjoy your life?

On the physical level, there are several energy-increasing effects that have been demonstrated with the use of WBV. Research has shown that WBV increases testosterone levels,[1] which are linked to greater energy for men and women, as well as heightened libido and sexual performance (see chapter 6). Circulation also improves, which provides more nutrients and oxygen to all cells producing energy. And as the exercise and workouts increase muscle strength, the whole body gains power and strength.

In the brain, WBV causes levels of the neurotransmitter serotonin to increase rapidly. High levels of serotonin improve sleep and promote a relaxed, happy, confident state of mind in which people are likely to be more active. Nothing saps your energy like depression and exhaustion, which can make just getting out of bed seem impossible.

WBV also works on the electromagnetic level (every time you are on a vibration plate, all your neurons are activated, shooting electromagnetic energy through your body and brain), and this electromagnetic energy is fundamentally connected to our physical and mental states. Norman Shealy, MD, PhD, founder of the American Holistic Medical Association and world-famous neurosurgeon, discusses this connection in his 2006 book *Soul Medicine:* "The body's electromagnetic field is a means through which biochemistry and physical anatomy interact with unseen energies. . . . In its component parts, and in its aggregate whole, our bodies, souls, minds, and emotional realms are interrelated energy systems. Energetic treatment of one part of this living matrix always affects the whole."[2]

"When I first started vibration therapy, I was so chronically fatigued that I would get a cart at the supermarket to lean on while I walked around, even if I only needed one item. After every vibration session (two per week), I felt stronger and energized; I was noticeably gaining vigor by the week. Two months into the therapy, there was a snowstorm that dropped a half a foot of snow overnight. I was late to my vibration appointment that day, because first I had to shovel out my driveway, and then I shoveled out my neighbor's driveway, as she is frail and elderly."

—Ellen Lehn, fifty-seven years old

"I had been vibrating just a few times when I went home after my three or four minutes of vibration, and I had so much energy I started scrubbing the kitchen floor by hand. When I finished with the floor, I started in on the walls. My husband, who was half asleep on the couch where we would usually both be after a long day at work, said to me, 'What has gotten into you?'"

—Anonymous

Life Force or Chi Energy

Western medicine recognizes that the nervous system is a pattern of electromagnetic signals—an EEG measures electronic brain waves, and an MRI creates images of the brain by measuring its electromagnetic energy. Quantum physics, meanwhile, describes the world of subatomic particles that makes up all matter and from which electromagnetic energy arises. Quantum physicist Ervin Lazlo explains that science is in the midst of a "shift from matter to energy as the primary reality. . . . There is no categorical divide between the physical world, the living world, and the world of mind and consciousness."[3] Shealy describes this connection: "A quantum universe is a set of probabilities, susceptible to influence by many factors, including thought, will, and intention."[4]

Many cultures throughout time have recognized the existence of a life-force energy. The Chinese call it chi, Indians call it prana, and European traditions have called it variously life force, soul, spirit, vital energy, vital principle, elan, and more. This energy guides and powers one's body and life, and disturbances in this energy due to trauma of any sort can have a profound effect on your physical and mental state.

Thousands of years ago, the Chinese discovered and mapped "energy meridians" in the body. Each of these energy pathways is associated with different organs and bodily systems. The Chinese medical system of acupuncture is based on maintaining a healthy and balanced flow of energy in those different meridians. Indian medicine describes chakras, spinning energy vortexes in our bodies, also associated with particular body systems and organs. In fact, some people can sense their own vibrational energy, and when these people stand on a vibrating plate, they report feeling energy shooting through their energy meridians and their chakras unblocking and spinning faster.

There is, in fact, measurable electromagnetic energy emanating from all things, because all substances are made from molecules that are, in turn, made from even smaller vibrating particles that have positive or negative electrical charges. Thus every substance has an electromagnetic charge that can be measured with sensitive scientific equipment. For example, Kirlian photography can detect and record the electromagnetic wavelengths around a person or object.[5]

Another energy-measuring system that is frequently used by medical doctors in Europe, where it was first developed in the 1950s, is called "electrodermal testing." This is a computer-linked testing system in which a probe that detects electromagnetic energy is touched to different acupuncture points on the hands and feet, and the energy in the associated energy meridian is graphed out on the computer screen.[6] With this system, one can instantly see which energy meridians, and thus their associated body organs or systems, are in balance, stressed (too much energy), or weakened (too little energy).

There are more than one hundred thousand such electrodermal screening machines in use worldwide, though very few are in the US where acceptance of energy medicine has been limited. There are many accounts of the detection of diseases, allergies, and toxic states using these machines.[7] One can also see, before spending a lot of time and money, which therapies or products resonate with an individual's electromagnetic energy and are therefore most likely to be successful. Electrodermal testing will also register changes in energy before and after vibration. In my natural health practice, where I regularly use both vibration and electrodermal testing, I have seen this many times.

Piezoelectricity?

On the physical level, WBV stimulates electromagnetic energy through a physical property of crystals called *piezoelectricity*—the ability of crystals to turn mechanical vibration into electrical vibration. Our bodies are living liquid crystals in the sense that we are highly organized molecular structures, and, as such, we have the property of piezoelectricity. Shealy describes our "bodies, souls, minds, and emotional realm" as a "living matrix" with the property of piezoelectricity.[8] "Waves of mechanical vibration moving through the living matrix produce electrical fields and vice versa. . . . Connective tissue is a liquid crystalline semiconductor. Piezoelectric signals from the cells can travel throughout the body in this medium."[9] The result is that "energetic treatment of one part of this living matrix always affects the whole."[10]

> *Every time you are on a vibration plate, your neurons fire, shooting electromagnetic energy through your body and brain . . . to heal, balance, and unblock your energy systems.*

Thus, every time you are on a vibration plate, your neurons fire, shooting electromagnetic energy through your body and brain, as your body turns the mechanical vibration into the electrical energy vibrations you need to heal, balance, and unblock your energy systems. Energy will flow into and through your energy meridians and chakra energy centers, increasing their proper spinning and energy flow. As these energy meridians and chakras are also linked to different organs, body systems, emotions, and needs, improving the flow of energy will help heal the physical body and mind, and improve life, all at the same time.

Pain Management

There are often rapid and dramatic decreases in pain for people using WBV, as is commonly seen with energy medicine. Acupuncture, for example, is well known for its ability to help with the reduction and management of pain. In fact, the American Academy of Pain Management, the largest organization of clinical pain practitioners in the world, reported in 1996 that the Shealy Institute, which Norman Shealy had founded twenty-five years earlier and where he uses primarily electromagnetic energy–medicine methods, has the best success of any pain clinic they have evaluated; and it does so at a cost that is 60 percent lower than the national average.[11]

Personally, I am very pain sensitive, usually requiring extra Novocain for the slightest dental procedure, but I once had a tooth pulled using only acupuncture (this was during a period when my chemical sensitivities were severe, and I could not tolerate any Western medicine drugs). Gripping the dental chair in great fear, to my amazement I only felt a wrenching, pulling sensation— no pain.

WBV is like acupuncture in its ability to stimulate our electromagnetic system.

WBV is like acupuncture in its ability to stimulate our electromagnetic system, and I have seen hundreds of people step on a Whole Body Vibration plate, and get off one to two minutes later with their pain gone. The placebo effect is unlikely, as many of these people have never heard of vibration or its benefits, and I usually don't have time at the crowded expos where this often happens to mention it before they step onto the plate.

Several research studies have also documented significant reductions in pain with WBV use. A 2011 study of twenty-three elderly subjects with knee osteoarthritis found an increase in function and decreases in self-reported pain, concluding that "whole-body vibration may represent a feasible and effective way of improving the functionality and self-perception of disease status in older adults with knee OA."[12]

Another study of fifty postmenopausal women with osteoporosis concluded that "whole-body vibration exercise using a Galileo machine [a low-intensity WBV machine] appears to be useful in reducing chronic back pain."[13] A third study, looking at sixty patients with chronic lower back pain during a six-month period concluded that "interestingly, well-controlled vibration may be the cure rather than the cause of lower back pain."[14]

Testimonials

"In 2008, according to the medical professionals, I needed both shoulders replaced. I was in a great deal of pain for years and was unable to raise my arms to reach anything above my head due to the pain and joint limitations. I had to modify all my exercise and drop cross-country skiing, mountain climbing, and yoga because of the pain and limited use of my shoulders and upper body. Depression from this limiting situation had me crying many days, as exercise and wellness had always been a huge part of my life. The pain was intense, twenty-four hours a day.

"Vibrating, in combination with eating well and an exercise program, has been a huge factor in lessening the twenty-four-hour pain I had in both shoulders. The shoulders still need replacing, but, because the pain is not bothering me, I can postpone the medical procedure."

—Wendy MacLean, small business co-owner

"I am a fifty-seven-year-old tradesman. After a lifetime of hard physical work, I had come to expect arthritic pain as a normal part of my workday. My ankles, knees, hips, and lower back jabbed at me constantly, and my response had been to tough it out. It was a losing proposition, and it appeared that hip replacement was inevitable.

"When a friend offered to let me try her vibration machine, the skeptic in me thought 'yeah, right.' That was weeks ago. This morning, I scampered down the stairs like a teenager. The remarkable thing is that I felt relief after the first five-minute session. Now, I simply stand on my WBV machine for five minutes each morning and head off to work with a happy song in my heart. The pain has gone. Imagine that."

—Wayne Young, master electrician

"When I first started working with Becky, about three months ago, I had constant pain in my right hip, right thigh, and both knees. I frequently walked with a limp, and climbing stairs was excruciatingly painful. In the last three months, I have made dramatic improvements. I was able to return to moderate exercising, and I have no pain in my hips or thighs. If anyone had told me that I could be so much stronger or that my pain could be reduced so much in such a brief period of time, I never would have believed it."

—Ann MacGibbon, PhD

chapter 6

Rejuvenation: Sex, Beauty, and Mobility

Feeling the Pain . . .

Oh my achin' joints!

Getting old is no picnic! Sex loses its appeal, beauty becomes an expensive full-time project, and mobility is a creaky, painful exercise of adjusting to limitations. But perhaps the fountain of youth does exist—and it vibrates! WBV has numerous global rejuvenation effects, such as raising human growth hormone and testosterone,[1] increasing circulation to all cells, detoxification, muscle and nerve stimulation, and energy balancing. These effects help your body repair its tissues and functions, and the effects can be especially dramatic with sexual libido and performance, skin tone and color, body shape, cellulite and fat deposits, and joint flexibility, pain, and strength.

Testosterone

WBV has been shown to increase levels of the sex hormone testosterone.[2] Normally, as men get older, their testosterone levels gradually decline—typically by about 1 percent per year after age thirty. Meanwhile, women have testosterone levels of about 10 percent of men's to begin with, and their testosterone levels drop rapidly at menopause. Testosterone, the major sex hormone for males, is closely linked to libido and sexual performance in men, as well as overall energy levels. Testosterone is also important for women.

WBV has been shown to increase levels of the sex hormone testosterone. . . . Testosterone, the major sex hormone for males, is closely linked to libido and sexual performance . . . , [and it] is also important for women.

Susan Rako, MD, a psychiatrist, wrote a groundbreaking book in 1996 called *The Hormone of Desire: The Truth about Testosterone, Sexuality, and Menopause* (updated in 1999, still in print, and still the most comprehensive and accurate body of information about the physiology and function of testosterone in women's bodies). In it she describes her experience, and the research, that has shown that testosterone levels affect libido (meaning one's "life force," not just sexual drive) for both men and women. In Dr. Rako's words, testosterone is "essential . . . to the healthy functioning of virtually all tissues in [a woman's] body, and to her experience of vital energy and sexual libido."[3] Typical high-testosterone effects include focused motivation, assertiveness, a sense of power, and enhanced sex drive. Healthy levels of testosterone help women take risks and live their lives with exuberance.

Testosterone also has powerful anti-aging effects. It turns fat into muscle, keeps skin supple, increases bone-mineral density, gives us a positive mood, and boosts our ability to handle stress. It supports mental health and cognitive functioning; also liver function and blood-vessel health. Low testosterone levels have been associated with heart attack, Alzheimer's disease, osteoporosis, and depression.

> **Testosterone is "essential . . . to the healthy functioning of virtually all tissues in [a woman's] body and to her experience of vital energy and sexual libido."**

There are drugs, such as Andro-gel, designed to raise testosterone in men, but as is generally true with prescription drugs, there are side effects[4] (and women and children must carefully avoid contact with these gels, or their hormone balances may be thrown off). The list of common side effects for men include nausea, vomiting, headache, dizziness, hair loss, trouble sleeping, change in sexual desire, redness/swelling of the skin, change in skin color, or acne.

Unlikely but serious side effects can also occur: breast pain/enlargement, swelling of the feet/ankles, weight gain, very slow/shallow/difficult breathing, weakness. And rare but very serious side effects include trouble urinating, mental/mood changes (e.g., depression, agitation, hostility), change in size/shape of the testicles, testicular pain/tenderness, stomach/abdominal pain, dark urine, change in the amount of urine, yellowing of eyes/skin, calf tenderness/swelling/pain. Why risk all this when there is a safe, natural approach that has many positive "side effects"?

While testosterone in the form of gels, creams, or pills are sometimes prescribed for women, the long-term safety of testosterone drug therapy for women is unknown. At this time, no commonly prescribed testosterone preparations have been approved by the Food and Drug Administration for use in women. If a testosterone drug is prescribed for women, it is off-label and not tested for safety.

WBV will not raise testosterone levels too high or too fast or interact negatively with other drugs or bodily functions. WBV promotes the body's ability to achieve its highest natural state of health. This is not to say that WBV is totally without risk. There are contraindications (see chapter 8), and it is important to understand detoxification and nutrition, but as a natural therapy, WBV promotes the optimal natural functioning of all body organs and systems.

Other WBV Effects
that Improve Libido and Sex

WBV also raises serotonin (see chapter 4), a neurotransmitter in the brain that is important for mood and the ability to experience pleasure, including sexual pleasure. Plus, confidence and a good mood go a long way toward improving sexual experiences. The increase in strength and physical energy levels associated with WBV will also help with sexual performance.

Another critical area affecting sexuality is your chi energy. Every time you are on a vibration plate, because of the piezoelectrical ability of the human body that converts mechanical vibration into electromagnetic energy (see chapter 5), you will be sending energy through the entire chakra system, and all of that energy will pass through the Kundalini chakra—the seat of your most basic survival needs, including sexual energy.

People who are sensitive to this energy can sometimes actually feel their chakras spinning. When these people stand on a vibrating plate, their eyes glaze over with delight, and they talk about feeling energy shooting through meridians, and chakras unblocking and spinning faster.

Whether people can identify "energy" or not, I have had some humorous situations develop when people try a vibration machine at expos. Some people end up suddenly feeling *very good indeed,* and the more uninhibited ones are not shy about expressing themselves. Strangers up and down the aisles turn to see what all the excitement, laughing, and oohs and ahs are about. Since this happens even with very gentle vibration where you cannot physically feel the vibration past your knees, and it happens quickly (in thirty to sixty seconds), it seems that at least some of this reaction is due to electromagnetic energy transmitting through the body, rather than hormonal or direct physical stimulation.

My favorite story of increasing libido and sexual enjoyment involves a middle-aged woman who came to me twice a week for three weeks. She was primarily interested in losing weight and increasing bone density. Her husband, though, was quite skeptical, "So, you think you are going to lose weight and increase bone density just by standing on that machine?!" After three weeks, my client came to me and said, "I think those hormonal affects you were talking about might be kicking in. . . . Now my husband says, '*Buy one.*'"

Beauty

Beauty is mostly health and happiness radiating through our bodies. Since WBV is fantastic for your physical and emotional health, you will be beautiful, too. Working out with vibration will tone your body, balance hormones, increase neurotransmitters in your brain, help you lose fat and cellulite, increase circulation to all tissues (resulting in increased collagen production which tightens and smooths skin), and put color in your cheeks and a sparkle in your eyes. When you feel good, you take better care of yourself: eating wisely, exercising more, maybe even sprucing up your wardrobe and changing your hair style. Then you get promoted at work, because now you're more effective and radiating confidence! It's like a snowball rolling downhill—it just keeps getting bigger and better all the time.

While cellulite and wrinkles are normal signs of aging, with improved health, they can be delayed and/or decreased. Cellulite is the lumpy appearance of fat that develops primarily in women, much to their annoyance, especially on the thighs, knees, backside, and upper arms. But cellulite is not really a fat problem, and it has nothing to do with how much you weigh. Cellulite is made up of a special type of fat, called "subcutaneous," that is within the skin layer, and it can't be burned as fuel, so you don't lose it by dieting.

As we age, circulation begins to decrease (especially to the thighs and other cellulite-prone areas) due to blood-vessel damage and the effects of decreasing estrogen. Poor circulation leads to a lack of nutrients and more toxins building up in the skin, which further damages blood vessels and lowers collagen production (the major component of a connective-tissue support structure that holds the subcutaneous fat in place). This all means that fat bulges out through the spaces between the fibers of that collagen-support structure, creating the lumpy effect. In other words, as one doctor put it, your backside is something like an old mattress with the stuffing bulging out!

Wrinkles are due to the loss of subcutaneous fat that, together with a healthy connective-tissue structure, usually plumps out and smooths skin, and the loss of elastin, which gives skin its flexibility, allowing it to stretch and give without damage.

WBV increases circulation, thus attacking the root cause of cellulite and wrinkles. Increased circulation brings more nutrients to the skin, causing greater collagen production, which strengthens the connective-tissue structure holding that unruly subcutaneous fat in place. Meanwhile, those nasty toxins and their associated free-radical damage are flushed out, further helping your skin to glow and retain its youthful appearance. WBV also increases human growth hormone (HGH), which promotes the healing of all tissues, including connective tissue and skin cells. Hop on a vibration machine, and you are fighting the "do not go gently into that good night" battle on all fronts.

WBV increases circulation, thus attacking the root cause of cellulite and wrinkles.

Add in good nutrition and nutritional supplements, and you have fresh troops pouring over the hills laden with supplies. Protein sources contain keratin, a building block for collagen and elastin, and antioxidants (fruits and vegetables) neutralize free-radical damage from toxins. Anti-aging creams are available now with these very ingredients incorporated into them, but keep in mind that nutrients are much more effectively absorbed into cells from the bloodstream than through the skin.

Also be sure to get plenty of potassium but low sodium (all fruits), for maintaining the proper electrolyte balance that promotes hydration of your cells, and lots of omega 3 oils to keep blood vessels and cell walls healthy. Together, these two factors insure good hydration to your cells; again, a more effective approach than hydrating the skin with lotions. Of course, you can always do both, lotions and nutrition, just don't forget the healthy food. As your mother said, "Eat your vegetables!"

Mobility

One of the most well-known and accepted uses of WBV is for physical therapy, about which entire books have been written.[5] WBV is used in physical therapy centers around the world. Sports franchises and top athletes use WBV for athletic training and to help the athletes heal faster from injuries, and they are less likely to be injured in the first place because their joints are stronger. WBV is effective therapy for a wide range of joint and movement issues, including arthritis, bursitis, tendonitis, fibromyalgia, pulled and strained muscles, weakness, range-of-motion issues, and poor flexibility.

WBV is effective therapy for a wide range of joint and movement issues.

One of the most obvious physical therapy benefits of WBV is that WBV combines strength training without stressing the joints, since you don't have to move on the vibration plate to work muscles. By holding different positions on the plate, you can target different muscles and joints (see chapter 1 for illustrations), and the intensity of the workout and stress on the joints can be adapted to varying levels of mobility, strength, and function.

Flexibility also increases, especially when stretching positions are used, due to the automatic reflex response causing rapid involuntary tightening and relaxing of muscles. Muscle fibers will automatically tense and relax at the same rate as the vibration, twenty to fifty times per second, and the relaxation phase of this response rapidly and gently increases flexibility.

The automatic reflex response has a massaging effect as well as a stretching effect that, along with relaxing tight muscles, increases circulation, bringing nutrients to the affected areas to aid in repair and regrowth. This massage effect happens automatically, but it can be heightened by placing the affected part of the body on the plate and relaxing. (One of my favorite positions, for pure enjoyment and relaxation, is a calf massage, where you lie down on your back, place your calves on the plate, cross your hands behind your head, and zone out.)

These stretching and massage effects can have rapid results. I have seen many people get on a machine and find that by the time they get off a few minutes later, painfully tight muscles have loosened, and they have a greater range of motion. Balance also improves, because specialized nerve clusters that control balance (called proprioceptors) are stimulated, along with the rest of the nervous system. This is of particular benefit to the elderly, who are at risk for dangerous falls.

Sometimes mobility problems are due to nerve issues, such as with multiple sclerosis, Parkinson's disease, and other conditions. Because WBV is calming, anti-inflammatory, and stimulates regeneration of the nervous system (see chapter 4), there can sometimes be dramatic results. One of my clients, Richard Hawkins, a retired orthopedic surgeon, had been a lifelong runner before he lost his ability to run due to a mysterious nerve issue. He had been in pain and unable to run for seven years when he met me. I suspected mercury poisoning, as he had been eating tuna fish every day for thirty years, and mercury is a potent neurotoxin. I suggested some heavy metal detox products, a few homeopathics, diet changes, and vibration. From the very first session of vibration (one minute), he noticed an improvement, and within a few weeks of twice-a-week, short sessions, he had begun to jog to his car with a big grin (see testimonial to follow).

Another important benefit of WBV is increased levels of HGH, which promote the healing of tissues critical for joint health and mobility along with all other tissues: ligaments, tendons, muscles, bones, and nerves. HGH levels typically fall with age, and any method of raising them is hotly pursued by those interested in athletic performance as well as simple daily pain relief and function.

Another important benefit of WBV is increased levels of HGH, which promote the healing of tissues critical for joint health and mobility.

Early research (2000) showed promising results with WBV, giving an increase in HGH levels of up to 150 percent.[6] More recent studies, however, have not delivered on this promise. A survey of recent WBV HGH research showed initial HGH gains with a first session of WBV but then a leveling off of gains. But, as with other WBV research on bone density and neurological diseases, these studies try to use too much vibration too quickly with elderly, fragile populations and without supporting detoxification and nutritional systems; thus they may not truly reflect the potential of WBV.

Pain and inflammation levels often drop rapidly using WBV, sometimes after just one session of one or two minutes (see also the Pain Management section in chapter 5). Such rapid reductions in pain and inflammation are likely due to WBV's effects on the electromagnetic system, as they happen too fast to attribute to other causes. To achieve lasting pain reduction, however, most people require regular sessions (usually two to three times per week) for at least a couple of months. But, like exercise, the ideal way to use WBV for continued lifelong health is to incorporate WBV into your life as a part of your daily routine. This is actually easy, since it is quick, feels great, and supplies instant gratification as well as long term benefits.

Pain and inflammation levels often drop rapidly using WBV, sometimes after just one session of one or two minutes.

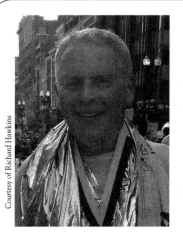

Courtesy of Richard Hawkins

"A lifelong runner, I gave up running at age sixty after developing numbness and pain in both feet. I spent seven years unable to run at all. I went to many different doctors, including specialists who told me there was nerve damage, and I would never get better, and I even tried surgery—all with no improvement. Then four years ago, I met Becky and started vibrating, increasing eventually to twenty minutes daily. I saw an improvement after the first session, and there has been a steady increase in function and feeling ever since. Now, four years later, I have just successfully completed this year's Boston Marathon, my twenty-seventh, at the age of seventy. Thanks, Becky!"

—Richard Hawkins, retired orthopedic surgeon

"As a division track and field athlete during college, I have endured many typical running injuries. More recently, while training for a half marathon, I suffered from a terrible bout of iliotibial band syndrome. Whole body vibration helped me to overcome this debilitating injury and complete the half marathon with a personal best (by nearly ten minutes!). I have also found that my recovery time after long runs has decreased dramatically while using vibration. Additionally, my strength and muscle tone have improved tremendously. I want to thank Becky for her commitment to and expertise in helping me to improve not only my athletic performance but my overall health."

—Hillary D. Repucci, nonprofit philanthropy

"I am in my seventies and a regular tennis player, but I have a shoulder injury from a bicycle accident years ago that never fully healed, and it has bothered me ever since. After only two weeks of vibration twice a week, it is getting a lot better. I would say it is 90 percent improved."

—Robert Williams, retired engineer

chapter 7

Detoxing with Whole Body Vibration

Toxins Everywhere

Our environment is loaded with toxins, and despite our best attempts to avoid them, some of these toxins will end up in our bodies. In a PBS television special several years ago, Bill Moyers, as a typical healthy person, had his blood tested at Mt. Sinai School of Medicine. Eighty-four different and highly toxic chemicals were found in his body.[1]

Once in our bodies, toxins may cause damage and disease. Toxins have been linked to almost all chronic health issues. Sherry A. Rogers, MD, a leading authority on environmental medicine, writes in her 2002 book, *Detoxify or Die*, "Pesticides, volatile organic hydrocarbons, auto and industrial pollution, mycotoxins, heavy metals, and more mimic any disease. They can cause any symptom or disease from high blood pressure, heart failure, osteoporosis, high cholesterol, arthritis, or Alzheimer's disease to fibromyalgia, degenerating disks, Parkinson's disease, depression, fatigue, irritable bowel, loss of libido, colitis, asthma, eczema, prostatitis, esophagitis, atrial fibrillation, GERD (gastroesophageal reflux disease), hearing loss, headaches, recurrent sinus, ear or throat infections, diabetes or cancer, and more."[2]

What Should One Do?

A regular detoxification program is a wise idea for everybody, and it is essential for people with chronic health issues. Remember, however, that detoxification should be done with caution, as detoxing is stressful for the body and can cause an increase in symptoms for someone with an already weakened body. Your body has natural systems to eliminate and neutralize toxins through the colon, liver, kidneys, lymphatic system, lungs, and skin. However, with the buildup of toxicity levels in your body and the consequent breakdown of health, it is important to support and aid your body in this process.

The muscle workout provided by WBV leads to an increased flow of the lymph moving toxins out of your body; [also the] increased circulation brings more nutrients and oxygen to all the cells.

A key benefit of vibration is that it is a powerful aid to your natural detoxification process. When vibrating, all your muscle fibers will involuntarily tense and relax at the same rate the machine is vibrating, twenty to fifty times per second. This creates a powerful massage for your lymphatic system, which is one of the body's primary natural detoxing tools. Unlike the heart and blood, this system does not have its own pumping system; muscles contracting around lymphatic vessels force the lymph (a clear fluid) to move. Thus the muscle workout provided by WBV leads to an increased flow of the lymph moving toxins out of your body. In addition, increased circulation brings more nutrients and oxygen to all the cells, helping them to function at a higher level and therefore dump more toxins and waste products into the lymphatic system.

Detox Overload

Detoxing with WBV is so powerful that it is the major limiting factor for most people using WBV—not muscle strength as many people assume. Detoxing will happen anytime you are on a machine, whether you just stand there or are actively exercising. As with detoxing after a massage or sauna or any other detox system, it is possible to overload your already-stressed detox pathways and have a temporary increase in symptoms. Common detox symptoms are exhaustion, headaches, and digestive problems, but any health issue that is linked to toxins can temporarily worsen as more toxins are released into the circulatory system. In fact, as any health problem you already have is a "weak link" in your system, when you stress your body with

Detox problems often do not show up until six to twenty-four hours after using WBV. So . . . use caution! too much detoxing, that weak link is a likely place to show the strain.

Candida yeast problems are also likely to flare up with detox overload. Since the liver is your major detox organ and also is part of the immune system, under the increased strain, your immune system may temporarily weaken, and this opportunistic parasite is likely to flare up. In fact, a Candida yeast flare up is a likely sign that you are in detox overload and need to do less vibration and possibly take a detox support supplement. Detox reactions are an enlightening opportunity to see the close connection between toxins and chronic health issues, something that is not always recognized by Western medicine.

Detox problems often do not show up until six to twenty-four hours after using WBV. So even though the vibration feels gentle and pleasant, use caution! Start slowly and increase slowly; many people will do best starting with just one minute on a gentle, low-power machine (see also chapter 8).

What to Do If You Experience Detox Overload

If any existing symptoms worsen, or new ones suddenly appear, it is possible that toxins are involved. You should stop vibrating, rest a few days, and, if symptoms decrease, you can start up again with less vibration. You can aid your body with detoxing by drinking extra water and/or juice to help flush out toxins and by getting plenty of sleep. Additionally, you can try any of the following:

- ◆ Activated charcoal: Take two to six capsules two to three times per day. Be sure to take this product on an empty stomach (one hour before food or two hours after food), because it will absorb nutrients as well as toxins.

- ◆ Modified citrus pectin: This comes in powder or capsule form, so take one scoop (or six capsules) once a day. This is a great product (sold under several different brand names; I usually use "PectaSol") that will be absorbed into your bloodstream, go everywhere in your body, and absorb only toxins. It can be taken with or without food.

- ◆ Protoclear: This is an excellent liver-supporting nutritional powder that combines many detox support nutrients, herbs, and PectaSol. Take one scoop once a day.

- ◆ Consult with a natural healthcare practitioner for your specific situation. Sometimes additional products and/or homeopathics are needed to resolve a situation.

Chapter 8

Choosing a Whole Body Vibration Machine

Of the many choices on the market, I have a current favorite, but I am always looking at and testing new machines, so check my website (www.BCVibrantHealth.com) for the latest information. I have seen over the last ten years, with myself and from working with hundreds of clients, that the type of machine you use is critical to the success of WBV. Since problems can develop from using the wrong machine (see below), I am very careful which WBV machines I use and recommend.

Double-Motor Vibration Machines

To achieve greater power, thus a greater workout effect, many WBV machines have two motors in them. However, as any engineer can attest, it is impossible to ever completely synchronize two motors. This lack of complete synchroniza-tion in the message sent through your nervous system and energy field by double-motor machines will have a desynchro-nizing effect on your nervous system and energy field, which can have very negative consequences over time. While people cannot detect the millisecond lack of synchronization on a conscious level while on a WBV machine, your nervous sys-tem and energy fields are extremely sensitive, and, on a deeper, unconscious level, they will be picking up this message.

Health effects from this desynchronization can be difficult to recognize and detect; since the athletes typically using this type of machine have such strong overall health, this subtle effect may go unnoticed for years. By the time trouble begins to develop (and since it involves the nervous system and energy fields, it can show up as any type of problem), these users have seen so many positive effects that they do not suspect vibration as being a factor.

Lack of complete synchronization in the message sent through your nervous system and energy field by double-motor machines will have a desynchronizing effect.

However, for me, as the sensi-tive canary in the mine, problems quickly become dramatic and very clear. After the first year with one of these double-motor machines, during which I did see improve-ments and became stronger than I had been in many years, my health suddenly deteriorated. I experienced a sudden and mysterious downturn and had such severe muscle weakness that I could not make it up the stairs or even across the room (this after climbing Mt. Washington only two weeks earlier), and my allergies, chemical sensitivities, multiple infections, digestive distress, and nervous system problems all returned. It was clear that it was linked to the vibration somehow, as I would get much worse after the slightest amount, but what exactly about the vibration was bothering me was difficult to determine.

After much trial and error, the problem was found to be the desynchronization effect of a double-motor machine. In fact, I only fully recovered when I began using a single-motor machine, which resynchronized my nervous system and chi energy. I have now been exclusively using single-motor machines for six years without a problem. The always perfectly synchronized message from these machines helps your system to synchronize itself while still providing all the other benefits of vibration.

Different Models and Makes

There are at least forty companies now making and selling vibration machines. Vibration machines were first developed (and are still best known) for their intense exercise capability. Many of these companies have the football mindset that the more power the better. Thus, many of the best-selling machines, and most of the machines you will find in health clubs and sports centers, are of the double-motor variety. Beyond this issue, there are several other variables to consider: direction of movement, frequencies, amplitudes, power (g force), durability, and cost. Read further for a more complete discussion of these factors, but the most important information for many people will be that you don't need to spend a great deal of money to get enormous benefit. There is a huge range of machines and you can get an effective and therapeutic machine for the price of a night in a nice hotel.

Direction of Movement

There are two major types of motion for vibration plates. Vertical, or linear, motion machines vibrate mostly up and down. This is the type of machine that I recommend for most people. As long as the vibration is produced with only one motor, this will provide a completely synchronized movement and message into your system, and this motion is the most stabilizing for your structural system.

Vertical, or linear, motion machines vibrate mostly up and down.

Very confusingly, variations of this first basic type of motion are produced by different motor configurations. The different motor types confer small amounts of horizontal motion and circular movement to the plate along with a predominantly vertical motion. To seem different (and better), companies come up with different names, such as three-dimensional, horizontal, spiral, circular, tri-planar, triangular, tri-phasic, multidimensional, omniflex, and piston. All these terms are describing basically the same type of motion.

There is, however, a great variation in amplitudes, g force, durability, and cost. (There are usually a range of frequency settings on any given machine, but not dramatic changes between machines.)

Amplitudes and frequency, thus the power (more technically referred to as gravitational force, or g force) of your vibration workout, can vary greatly. To get a sense of what I mean by g force, imagine putting your hand on a purring cat versus a jack

A second major type of vibration machine utilizes oscillation across a fulcrum in the middle of the plate, so that the plate rises and falls on either side like a child's seesaw.

hammer—these are very different experiences because of the different amplitudes and frequencies of the vibrations. A jack-hammer's amplitude of vibration is much greater than a cat's purr, so even though the frequency of the cat's purr is greater, the total g force, and effect, is greater for the jack hammer. (See the next page for details.)

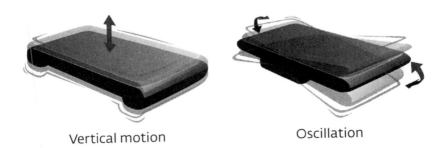

Vertical motion   Oscillation

A second major type of vibration machine utilizes oscillation across a fulcrum in the middle of the plate, so that the plate rises and falls on either side like a child's seesaw. This motion is called oscillation, pivotal, or teeter-totter. These machines usually have greater amplitudes (up to 10 mm) but lower frequencies. They can provide a good workout for less cost. However, for total health, I recommend a single motor vertical vibration machine with its perfect synchronization and gentler motion. Too much vibration is much more of a problem than too little vibration. If someone is determined to use oscillation vibration, I would recommend that he also do at least an equal amount of time on a single motor linear vibration machine.

In fact, there are now machines that have both types of motion available in one machine, and each is independently controlled. These machines are described as "dual motion" or "hybrid." Don't confuse dual *motion* with dual *motor*. Dual motor refers to two motors operating at the same time, and I recommend you always avoid this type of vibration (see above). Dual motion machines have two motors and two motions, often with the option of operating both at the same time—don't do that! As long as only one motor is operating at a time, this is a viable option, though not my highest recommendation.

The final type of machine is one in which a linear vibration motion is generated by sonic (sound) waves. No actual sound is produced by these machines; the term "sonic" is used here to describe a sound wave–type of mechanism that produces a vertical movement—not a sound. These machines typically can create very powerful vibrations, but the cost is also very high

($8,000–$15,000) without adding significant benefits. These machines can generate very high amplitudes and g forces.

Remember that intense exercise is only one of many benefits you can get from vibration. For many people, if they try to work out too intensely with vibration at the beginning, they will end up feeling worse instead of better because of too much detoxing. Be patient! Remember that you can get exercise many ways. The workout effect is not the only benefit, and it is not what makes vibration so unique. Muscle strength, toning, and weight loss are only the tip of the iceberg when it comes to vibration's benefits.

Gravitational (g) Force, Amplitude, and Frequency

The power of a machine (g force) is determined by the amplitude (the distance the plate moves) and the frequency (the rate or speed of vibration).[1] The greater the amplitude and the frequency, the greater the g force. Changing the amplitude dramatically changes the g force; that is, the purring cat (low amplitude) versus the jack hammer (high amplitude). To change the amplitude significantly, one often needs to change machines.

Amplitude can range from less than 1 mm (0.3 maximum g force) for very gentle, low-power, vertical-motion machines to

---

[1] G force is also affected by mass; in this situation, the weight of the person standing on the plate. Since companies don't use a standard weight to determine g force, this is not an exact way to compare machines, but it can still be a useful measure to bear in mind. G force is measured and expressed in g units, which for simplicity will be implied but not written out in this book. For example, 0.3 g maximum g force becomes 0.3 maximum g force.

2.5 mm (2.65 maximum g force) for the most powerful single-motor machines currently available. Double-motor, linear-motion machines can deliver higher amplitudes and g forces (up to 4 mm and 15 g), but as noted earlier, I don't recommend these machines. Oscillating motion machines have higher amplitudes (up to 11 mm), but since the motion is so intense, the frequency is lower, resulting in 5 to 7 maximum g forces.

Sonic vibration machines can have amplitudes up to 27 mm. These are huge amplitudes that might vibrate you right off the plate if the frequency weren't automatically set to be low. These machines create very high g forces of 18—that, unless you are training to be an astronaut, are totally unnecessary.

The frequency is the rate at which a machine vibrates, and most machines have a wide range of frequency (speed) settings. Linear vibration machines have settings ranging from 20–50 Hz (vibrations per second). Oscillation machines typically have lower frequency ranges (5–30 Hz) because of the higher amplitudes.

Much effort has gone into figuring out which frequencies are the best for losing weight and cellulite, increasing bone density and muscle strength, etc. My experience is that focusing on exactly what frequency is the best for achieving certain effects is usually a moot point. For the average person, the detoxing effect is the major limiting factor; therefore, you should start at the lowest speed and increase slowly. It is great to work your way up to the higher frequencies, and they do have more powerful effects, but you have to go slowly, or you may end up disappointed and stop entirely!

Plus, all vibration has huge effects on all parts of your body, so no matter what frequency you use, you will be on your way to achieving the desired results. When you have worked your way up and can tolerate the higher frequencies, you may choose to optimize muscle strengthening by working out at 35 Hz or achieve greater muscle massage, lymph drainage, and neurological stimulation at 40–50 Hz.

Durability

This depends on the quality of construction. Plastic parts are not as durable as steel, but for low-cost, low–g force machines, plastic can be a reasonable option. Larger, more powerful machines are usually made of steel. Many machines are made overseas and shipped to the US. Quality can vary widely, so be sure to check the warranty terms and weight limits.

Cost

There is an enormous range in the cost of machines. You can spend anywhere from $150 for a gentle vertical vibration machine to $15,000 for a sonic vibration machine. The cost depends on many factors, including the type of machine and amount of power, the quality of construction, availability of knowledgeable customer support services, demand, and the marketing strategy.

Generally, the higher the g force and amplitude of a machine, the larger, heavier, and more expensive it is likely to be. This is because the motor must be more powerful to generate the greater amplitude, and since vibration tends to shake things apart, the machine must be built to withstand increasing force. See "Five Levels of Vibration Machines" on the next page for a more detailed breakdown, and keep in mind when choosing a machine that more power does not mean better! The machines I most often recommend are $150 to $1,000. See my website for my latest recommendations.

Guidelines for Choosing Your Vibration Machine

These guidelines refer to the categories listed below, where I have separated vertical vibration machines into five levels based on the power, or gravitational force. The guidelines are not meant to be a substitute for a medical doctor's evaluation and advice. Before starting any exercise program, you should consult with your doctor.

More power does not mean better! The machines I most often recommend are $150 to $1,000.

First, make sure you do not have any of the contraindications for using WBV (see pages 87–89). Then assess your overall health, as your ability to tolerate detoxing, thus vibration, depends on the state of your health and the level of toxins stored in your body. These factors are very important in choosing a machine and in how rapidly you will be able to increase the amount of WBV you do. I highly recommend discussing your options with a qualified WBV specialist. Remember, everyone is unique, and these are general guidelines only.

Five Levels of Vibration Machines

Level 1—Extremely Gentle: Amplitudes of less than or equal to 1 mm and maximum g forces of less than 1.0. These machines are extremely gentle and can be suitable for the very ill, the weak, or the elderly. If a person can tolerate more vibration, I would recommend a greater g force machine. I have seen prices ranging from $450 to $3,000 (perhaps high because demand has been low).

Level 2—Gentle: Amplitudes of 1–1.5 mm and 1–1.5 maximum g force. This gentle but therapeutic vibration is suitable for older people and those with health issues, and there are good, inexpensive options ($150–$1,000). The disadvantages are that they do not offer much of a workout and may not be as durable (depending on construction) as machines built to withstand greater vibration. They are highly therapeutic for the internal organs, the nervous system, and chi energy, but a longer amount of time is needed on these machines for increasing bone density.

Level 3—Strong but Gentle: Mid-range power (1.5–2 mm amplitude, 1.5–2.3 maximum g force) and available at reasonable prices ($1,000–$3,000). These machines usually feature durable metal construction, are therapeutic for internal systems and the nervous system, and offer an effective workout and bone density stimulus while still having a gentle vibration. Be sure it uses only a single motor. These machines offer a good workout and are highly beneficial for many health issues. They may be too strong a vibration for fragile or ill people.

NOTE: I have lately seen double-motor machines listed with 12–15 maximum g forces but also advertised as having only 2–3 mm amplitudes. I doubt the accuracy of this, especially as I used to see these same machines listed with 4–5 mm amplitudes.

Level 4—Powerful: I have found a relatively powerful but still single-motor vibration machine (2.5 mm amplitude, 2.65 maximum g force) that gives a major workout and bone-building stimulus. These machines are suitable for athletes and young and otherwise strong, healthy people. They are more expensive ($3,500–$5,500) but very durable.

Level 5—Extremely Powerful: Linear motion machines with a maximum g force greater than 3 are usually double-motor machines, and the prices are usually quite high ($2,000–$15,000). I do not recommend these machines. Some professional athletes insist on double-motor machines, thinking they need the extra power. I disagree and have heard of preliminary studies showing that athletic performance increases more with single motor vibration than with double motor, possibly because the complete synchronization in the single leads to extra coordination, balance, and response times. If you must use a double-motor system, spend at least an equal amount of time on a single-motor system to protect yourself. Oscillation machines can deliver high g forces at a low cost ($200–$2,000), but again I would recommend using an equal amount of vertical vibration.

Getting Started

Increasing the frequency intensifies the experience more rapidly than just increasing the length of time you are on the machine. A good way to start is with one minute at the lowest speed, increasing only one minute per day (or less) until you get an idea of how your body responds to vibration, until you can tolerate up to ten to twenty minutes. Then increase the frequency by one setting, but drop the time back to just a few minutes and slowly work your way up again as before.

Start with one minute at the lowest speed, increasing only one minute per day (or less), until you can tolerate up to ten to twenty minutes.

If you find that you are not having any problems and you just feel great, try to up your time at a faster pace. But if you are having problems of any sort, stop vibrating altogether, and see if you get better. There is a huge range of how people respond to vibration. A healthy young athlete might be able to jump on a powerful machine and do ten minutes and feel great the first time he ever uses one. Other people, those with health issues, may need months just to get to ten minutes on a low-power machine.

For improving the general health and well-being for people with chronic health issues, the goal is to gradually increase the time of vibration to at least ten minutes per day at a mid-range frequency on a level 2 "gentle" machine. This amount of WBV will supply a big dose of the many benefits every day.

People in better health and those looking to increase bone density ideally would use a level 3 or 4 machine, but if the cost, or detoxing effect, is too much for them, a level 2 machine will still deliver great benefits. For healthy athletic types, at least ten minutes of exercise per day on a level 3 or 4 machine at 35 Hz is recommended. Even with the proper machines, do not do more than sixty minutes of low-amplitude vibration or twenty minutes of higher amplitude vibration per day.

The sooner you start a natural health regimen the better!

Keep in mind that any vibration can have dramatic positive effects, so start slowly. Increase at your own pace, and enjoy!

Some people with severe health issues and weak constitutions may not be able to tolerate any vibration at all. These people should use other natural health remedies, such as nutritional supplements, acupuncture, and chiropractic to build up their strength before incorporating WBV. The sooner you start a natural health regimen the better! It is always easier to address a health issue before it becomes serious; prevention is easier than repair!

There is a huge range of ability to tolerating vibration. For example, I had a sixty-year-old client with chronic fatigue and depression who experienced a dramatic improvement in energy and mood after his first one-minute session at the lowest frequency on a "gentle" machine. He bought the machine and was able to increase to ten minutes at the highest frequency (50 Hz) within two months. At the other end of the spectrum is myself. I've been at this for six years and have supplemented with an impressive number of nutritional products and other types of natural health therapies. I am still not at the highest settings on my "gentle" machine, but that's not the goal. The goal is to feel great, and I do!

Contraindications[1]

It is always advisable to consult with your physician before starting any exercise program. Ongoing research in the field of Whole Body Vibration (WBV) indicates that many people can benefit from this form of exercise. However, if you suffer from any of the following contraindications, it is imperative that you discuss WBV therapy with your physician before beginning any training program with WBV equipment.

Please do not use any WBV device without first getting approval from your doctor if you have any of the following:

Relative contraindications—meaning that with special care and treatment, these conditions can sometimes not be a hindrance to, and may even benefit from, WBV.

- ◆ pregnancy
- ◆ epilepsy
- ◆ gallstones, kidney stones, bladder stones
- ◆ articular rheumatism, arthrosis
- ◆ acute rheumatoid arthritis
- ◆ heart failure
- ◆ cardiac dysrhythmias

- cardiac disorders (post-myocardial infarction [heart attack])

- metal or synthetic implants (e.g., pacemaker, artificial cardiac valves, recent stents, or brain implants)

- chronic back pain (after fracture, disc disorders, or spondylosis)

- severe diabetes mellitus with peripheral vascular disease or neuropathy

- tumors (excluding metastases in the musculoskeletal system)

- spondylolisthesis without gliding

- movement disorders, Parkinson's disease

- chondromalacia of the joints of the lower extremities, osteonecrosis

- arterial circulation disorders

- venous insufficiency with ulcus cruris

- Morbus Sudeck Stadium II (or complex regional pain syndrome [CRPS])

- lymphatic edema

- postoperative wounds

Absolute contraindications—meaning **do not use** any WBV device at all if you have any of the following *or if you have any concerns about your physical health!*

- acute inflammations, infections, and/ or fever

- acute arthropathy or arthrosis

- acute migraine
- fresh (surgical) wounds
- implants of the spine
- acute or chronic deep vein thrombosis or other thrombotic afflictions
- acute disc-related problems, spondylosis, gliding spondylolisthesis, or fractures
- severe osteoporosis with BMD less than 70 mg/ml
- spasticity (after stroke, spinal cord lesion, etc.)
- Morbus Sudeck Stadium I (CRPS I)
- tumors with metastases in the musculoskeletal system
- vertigo or positional dizziness
- acute myocardial infarction

Endnotes

Chapter 2

1. C. Bosco et al., "Hormonal Responses to Whole-Body Vibration in Men," *European Journal of Applied Physiology* 81 (2000): 449–454.

2. D. Vissers et al., "Effect of Long-Term Whole Body Vibration Training on Visceral Adipose Tissue: A Preliminary Report." *Obes Facts* 3, no. 2 (2010): 93–100.

3. Gina Kolata, "Low Buzz May Give Mice Better Bones and Less Fat." *New York Times* 30 (October 30, 2007), accessed January 1, 2013, http://tinyurl.com/7wjq8xq.

Chapter 3

1. "Good Vibrations: A New Treatment under Study by NASA-Funded Doctors Could Reverse Bone Loss Experienced by Astronauts in Space," NASA, accessed January 1, 2013, https://web.archive.org/web/20020209180125/http://science.nasa.gov/headlines/y2001/ast02nov_1.htm.

2. Ibid.

3. Kolata, "Low Buzz May Give Mice Better Bones and Less Fat."

4. A. Prioreschi, T. Oosthuyse, I. Avidon, and J. McVeigh, "Whole Body Vibration Increases Hip Bone Mineral Density in Road Cyclists." *Int J Sports Med.* 33, no. 8 (August 2012): 593–9, accessed January 1, 2013, doi:10.1055/s-0032-1301886.

5. Joseph Mercola, DO, "Vibrational Training Beats Weight Training for Building Stronger, Denser Bones," accessed January 1, 2013, http://fitness .mercola.com/sites/fitness/archive/2012/11/23/power-plate-training-for-afi-bromyalgia.aspx?e_cid=20121123_DNL_art_1.

6. R. W. Lau et al., "The Effects of Whole Body Vibration Therapy on Bone Mineral Density and Leg Muscle Strength in Older Adults: A Systematic Review and Meta-Analysis," *Clin Rehabil* 25, no. 11 (November 2011): 975–88, accessed January 1, 2013, doi:10.1177/0269215511405078.

7. Kolata, "Low Buzz May Give Mice Better Bones and Less Fat."

8. Lara Pizzorno, MA, LMT, and Jonathan V. Wright, MD, *Your Bones: How You Can Prevent Osteoporosis and Have Strong Bones for Life—Naturally* (Mount Jackson, VA: Praktikos Books, 2011), 6.

9. Ibid., 17–23.

10. Ibid., 31–40.

11. Ibid., 134.

12. Ibid., 67.

13. Ibid., 165.

14. Bruce West, DC, "Osteoporosis and How to Heal Bones," *Health Alert* 17, no. 6 (2006).

Chapter 4

1. Gretchen Reynolds, "Jogging Your Brain," *New York Times* magazine, (April 2012): 46.

2. M. Ariizumi and A. Okada, "Effect of Whole Body Vibration on the Rat Brain Content of Serotonin and Plasma Corticosterone," *Eur J Appl Physiol Occup Physiol* 52, no. 1 (1983): 15–9.

3. B. del Pozo-Cruz et al., "Using Whole-Body Vibration Training in Patients Affected with Common Neurological Diseases: A Systematic Literature Review," *J Altern Complement Med* 18, no. 1 (January 2012): 29–41.

4. G. Ebersbach, D. Edler, O. Kaufhold, and J. Wissel, "Whole Body Vibration versus Conventional Physiotherapy to Improve Balance and Gait in Parkinson's Disease," *Arch Phys Med Rehabil* 89, no. 3 (March 2008): 399–403.

Chapter 5

1. C. Bosco et al., "Hormonal Responses to Whole-Body Vibration in Men," 449–454.

2. Norman Shealy, MD, PhD, *Soul Medicine* (Santa Rosa, CA: Elite Books, 2006), 208–212.

3. Ibid., 16.

4. Ibid.

5. Richard Gerber, MD, *Vibrational Medicine*, 3rd ed. (Rochester, NY: Bear and Co., 2001), 53–56.

6. American Association of Acupuncture and Bio-Energetic Medicine, "Basic Explanation of the Electrodermal Screening Test and the Concepts of Bio-Energetic Medicine," http://www.healthy.net/scr/article.aspx?Id=1085.

7. Shealy, *Soul Medicine*, 206.

8. Ibid., 212.

9. Ibid., 213.

10. Ibid., 212.

11. Ibid., 45.

12. N. C. Avelar, et al., "The Effect of Adding Whole-Body Vibration to Squat Training on the Functional Performance and Self-Report of Disease Status in Elderly Patients with Knee Osteoarthritis: A Randomized, Controlled Clinical Study. *J Altern Complement Med* 17, no. 12 (December 2011): 1149–55, doi: 10.1089/acm.2010.0782.

13. J. Iwamoto, T. Takeda, Y. Sato, and M. Uzawa, "Effect of Whole-Body Vibration Exercise on Lumbar Bone Mineral Density, Bone Turnover, and Chronic Back Pain in Post-Menopausal Osteoporotic Women Treated with Alendronate," *Aging Clin Exp Res* 17, no. 2 (April 2005): 157–63.

14. J. Rittweger, J. Karsten, K. Kautzsch, P. Reeg, and D. Felsenberg, "Treatment of Chronic Lower Back Pain with Lumbar Extension and Whole Body Vibration Exercise in a Randomized Controlled Trial," *Spine* 27, no. 17 (2002): 1829–1834.

Chapter 6

1. C. Bosco et al., "Hormonal Responses to Whole-Body Vibration in Men," 449–454.

2. Ibid.

3. Susan Rako, MD, *The Hormone of Desire: The Truth about Testosterone, Sexuality, and Menopause*, (New York: Three Rivers Press, 1996), 25.

4. http://www.rxlist.com/androgel-side-effects-drug-center.htm.

5. Alfio Albasini, Martin Krause, and Ingo Volker Rembitzki, *Using Whole Body Vibration in Physical Therapy and Sport: Clinical Practice and Treatment Exercises* (Edinburgh; New York: Churchill Livingstone/Elsevier, 2010).

6. C. Bosco et al., "Hormonal Responses to Whole-Body Vibration in Men," 449–454.

Chapter 7

1. "Chemical Body Burden," http://www.pbs.org/tradesecrets/problem /bodyburden.html.

2. Sherry A. Rogers, MD, *Detoxify or Die* (Sarasota, FL: Sand Key Co., 2002), 89.

Chapter 8

1. http://www.bodyvibeusa.com/Contraindications.aspx.

Additional
Research Studies

For even more information, go to http://www.ncbi.nlm.nih
.gov/pubmed and use the search string "whole body vibration"
to find hundreds of other research studies.

Performance

Bosco C., M. Cardinale, R. Colli, J. Tihanyi, S. P. von Duvillard, and A. Viru.
"The Influence of Whole Body Vibration on the Mechanical Behavior of
Skeletal Muscle." *Clinical Physiology* 19 (1999): 183–187.

Bosco C., M. Cardinale., and O. Tsarpela. "Influence of Vibration on
Mechanical Power and Electromyogram Activity in Human Arm Flexor
Muscles." *European Journal of Applied Physiology* 79 (1999): 306–311.

Bosco C., M. Cardinale, O. Tsarpela, and E. Locatelli. "New Trends in Training Science: The Use of Vibrations for Enhancing Performance." *New
Studies in Athletics* 4, no. 14 (1999): 55–62.

Bosco, C., R. Colli, E. Introini, M. Cardinale, O. Tsarpela, A. Madella, J.
Tihanyi, and A. Viru. "Adaptive Responses of Human Skeletal Muscle to
Vibration Exposure." *Clinical* Physiology 19 (1999): 183–187.

de Ruiter, C. J., R. M. van der Linden, M. J. A. van der Zijden, A. P. Hollander, and A. de Haan. "Short-Term Effects of Whole-Body Vibration on Maximal Voluntary Isometric Knee Extensor Force and Rate of Force Rise." *European Journal of Applied Physiology* 88 (2003): 472–475.

Hinman, M. "Whole Body Vibration: A New Exercise Approach." Department of Physical Therapy. The University of Texas Medical Branch.

Humphries, B., and G. Warman. "The Assessment of Vibromyographical Signals in the Time and Frequency Domains during a Fatigue Protocol." The School of Health and Human Performance, Central Queensland University.

Issurin, V. B., and G. Tenenbaum. "Acute and Residual Effects of Vibratory Stimulation on Explosive Force in Elite and Amateur Athletes." *Journal of Sports Sciences* 17 (1999): 177–182.

Mester, J. "Knocken und Muskel, neue Welte, Vibrationsbelastung und Vibrationstraining im Spitzensport, Interdisciplinair Kongress mit Workshop: Radiologische Osteoporosediagnostik." Berlin, 2001.

Nishihihira, Y., T. Iwasaki, A. Hatta, T. Wasaka, T. Kaneda, K. Kuroiwa, S. Akiyama, T. Kida, and K.S. Ryol. "Effect of Whole Body Vibration Stimulus and Voluntary Contraction on Motoneuron Pool." Japan Society of Exercise and Sports Physiology, Tsukuba (2002): 83–86.

Rittweger, J., G. Beller, and D. Felsenberg. "Acute Physiological Effects of Exhaustive Whole-Body Vibration Exercise in Man." *Clinical Physiology* 20 (2000): 134–142.

Rittweger, J., J. Ehrig, K. Just, M. Mutschelknauss, and K. A. Kirsch. "Oxygen Uptake in Whole-Body Vibration Exercise Influence of Vibration Frequency, Amplitude, and External Load." *International Journal of Sports Medicine* 23 (2002): 428–432.

Rittweger, J., M. Mutschelknauss, and D. Felsenberg. "Acute Changes in Neuromuscular Excitability after Exhaustive Whole Body Vibration Exercise as Compared to Exhaustion by Squatting Exercise." *Clinical Physiology and Functional Imaging* 23, no. 2 (2003): 81–86.

Rittweger, J., H. Schiessl, and D. Felsenberg. "Oxygen Uptake during Whole Body Vibration Exercise Comparison with Squatting as a Slow Voluntary Movement." *European Journal of Applied Physiology* 86 (2001): 169–173.

Torvinen, S., P. Kannus, H. Sievänen, T. A. H. Järvinen, M. Pasanen, S. Kontulainen, T. L. N. Järvinen, M. Järvinen, P. Oja, and I. Vuori. "Effect of Four-Month Vertical Whole Body Vibration on Performance and Balance." *Medicine and Science in Sports and Exercise* 34, no. 9 (2002): 1523–1528.

———. "Effect of Vibration Exposure on Muscular Performance and Body Balance: Randomized Cross-Over Study." *Clinical Physiology and Functional Imaging* 22 (2002): 145–152.

Quality of Life

Hormonal Response

Bosco, C., M. Jacovelli, O. Tsarpela, M. Cardinale, M. Bonifazi, J. Tihanyi, M. Viru, A. de Lorenzo, and A. Viru. "Hormonal Responses to Whole-Body Vibration In Men." *European Journal of Applied Physiology* 81 (2000): 449–454.

Cardinale, M. "The Effects of Vibration on Human Performance and Hormonal Profile." The Semmelweis University Doctoral School, Faculty of Physical Education and Sport Sciences, Budapest (2002).

Cardinale, M., and J. Lim. "Electromyography Activity of Vastus Lateralis Muscle during Whole-Body Vibrations of Different Frequencies." *Journal of Strength and Conditioning Research* 17, no. 3 (2003): 621–624.

Carroll, T. J., S. Riek, and R. G. Carson. "Neural Adaptation Induced by Resistance Training in Humans." *Journal of Physiology* 544, no.2 (2002): 641–652.

Delecluse, C., M. Roelants, and S. Verschueren. "Strength Increase after Whole Body Vibration Compared with Resistance Training." *Official Journal of the American College of Sports Medicine* (2003): 1033–1041.

Giunta, M., M. Cardinale, F. Agosti, A. Patrizi, E. Compri, A. E. Rigamonti, and A. Sartorio. "Growth Hormone-Releasing Effects of Whole Body Vibration Alone or Combined with Squatting Plus External Load in Severely Obese Female Subjects." *Obes Facts* 5, no. 4 (2012): 567–74. doi:10.1159/000342066.

Sartorio, A., F. Agosti, A. De Col, N. Marazzi, F. Rastelli, S. Chiavaroli, C. L. Lafortuna, S. G. Cella, and A. E. Rigamonti. "Growth Hormone and Lactate Responses Induced by Maximal Isometric Voluntary Contractions and Whole-Body Vibrations in Healthy Subjects." *J Endocrinol Invest* 34, no. 3 (March 2011): 216–21. doi:10.3275/7255.

Blood Circulation

Kerschan-Schindl, K., S. Grampp, C. Henk, H. Resch, E. Preisinger, V. Fialka-Moser, and H. Imhof. "Whole-Body Vibration Exercise Leads to Alterations in Muscle Blood Volume." *Clinical Physiology* 21 (2001): 377–382.

Pain Management

Brumagne, S., P. Cordo, R. Lysens, S. Verschueren, and S. Swinnen. "The Role of Paraspinal Muscle Spindles in Lumbosacral Position Sense in Individuals with and without Low Back Pain." *Spine* 25, no. 8(2000): 989–994.

Gianutsos, J. G., J. H. Ahn, L. C. Oakes, E. F. Richter, B. B. Grynbaum, and H. G. Thistle. "The Effects of Whole Body Vibration on Reflex-Induced Standing in Persons with Chronic and Acute Spinal Cord Injury." New York School of Medicine at the AAPMR (2000).

Bone Density

Bruyere, O., M. A. Wuidart, E. di Plama, M. Gourlay, O. Ethgen, F. Richy, and J. Y. Reginster. "Presentation: Controlled Whole Body Vibrations Improve Health Related Quality of Life in Elderly Patients." American College of Rheumatology. (October 23–28, 2003): Abstract 1271.

Falempin, M., and S. F. In-Albon. "Influence of Brief Daily Tendon Vibration on Rat Soleus Muscle in a Non-weight Bearing Situation." *Journal of Applied Physiology* 87, no. 1 (1999): 3–9.

Flieger, J., T. Karachalios, L. Khaldi, P. Raptou, and G. Lyritis. "Mechanical Stimulation in the Form of Vibration Prevents Postmenopausal Bone Loss in Ovariectomized Rats." *Calcified Tissue International* 63 (1998): 510–514.

Rubin, C., M. Pope, C. Fritton, M. Magnusson, and K. McLeod. "Transmissibility of 15-Hz to 35-Hz Vibrations to the Human Hip and Lumbar Spine: Determining the Physiologic Feasibility of Delivering Low-Level Anabolic Mechanical Stimuli to Skeletal Regions at Greatest Risk of Fracture because of Osteoporosis." *Spine* 28, no. 23 (2003): 2621–2627.

Rubin, C., R. Recker, D. Cullen, J. Ryaby, J. McCabe, and K. McLeod. "Prevention of Postmenopausal Bone Loss by a Low Magnitude, High-Frequency Mechanical Stimuli: A Clinical Trial Assessing Compliance, Efficacy, and Safety." *Journal of Bone and Mineral Research* 19, no. 3 (2004): 343–351.

Rubin, C., S. A. Turner, S. Bain, C. Mallinckrodt, and K. McLeod. "Anabolism: Low Mechanical Signals Strengthen Long Bones." *Nature* 412 (2001): 603–604.

Rubin, C., G. Xu, and S. Judex. "Anobolic Activity of Bone Tissue, Suppressed by Disuse, Is Normalized by Brief Exposure to Extremely Low Magnitude Mechanical Stimuli." *FASEB Journal* 15 (2001): 2225–2229.

Schiessel, H., H. M. Frost, and W. S. S. Jee. "Estrogen and Bone-Muscle Strength and Mass Relationships." *Bone* 22, no. 1 (1998): 1–6.

van Loon, J. W. A., J. P. Veldhuijzen, and E. H. Burger. "Bone and Spaceflight: An Overview." In *Biological and Medical Research in Space*, edited by D. Moore, P. Bie, and H. Oser, 259–299. Berlin Heidelberg: Springer-Verlag, 1996.

Verschueren, S., M. Roelants, R. Delecluse, S. Swinnen, D. Vanderschueren, and S. Boonen. "Effects of 6-Month Whole Body Vibration Training on Hip Density, Muscle Strength, and Postural Control in Postmenopausal Women: A Randomized Controlled Pilot Study." *Journal of Bone and Mineral Research* 19, no. 3 (2004): 352–359.

Metabolism

Frank, H., B. Moos, A. Kaufmann, and H. A. Herber. "Anti-Cellulite Untersuchung. Sanaderm, Fach klinik fur Hautkrankheiten. *Allergologie* (2003): 1–35.

Flexibility/Mobility/Balance

Ishitake, T., Y. Miyazaki, H. Ando, and T. Mataka. "Suppressive Mechanism of Gastric Mobility by Whole Body Vibration." *International Arch. Occup. Environ. Health* 72 (1999): 469–474.

Miyamoto, K., S. Mori, S. Tsuji, S. Tanaka, M. Kawamoto, T. Mashiba, S. Komatsubara, T. Akiyama, J. Kawanishi, and H. Norimatsu. "Whole Body Vibration Exercise in Elderly People." *IBMS-JSBMR* (2003): Abstract P506.

Rauch, F., and J. Rittweger. "What Is New in Neuro-Musculoskeletal Interactions? *Journal Musculoskeletal Neuron Interactions* 2, no. 5 (2002): 1–5.

Runge, M. "Therapiemöglichkeiten bei Harninkontinenz; überwinden des Tabu." *Der Hausarzt* 2 (2002): 56–61.

Runge, M., G. Rehfeld, and E. Reswick. "Balance Training and Exercise in Geriatric Patients. *Journal of Musculoskeletal Interactions* 1 (2000): 54–58.

Slavko, R., R. Hilfiker, K. Herren, L. Radlinger, and E. D. de Bruin. "Effects of Whole-Body Vibration on Postural Control in the Elderly: A Systematic Review and Meta-Analysis." BMC Geriatrics 11, no. 72 (2011). The electronic version of this article can be found online at www.biomed central.com/1471-2318/11/72, doi:10.1186/1471-2318-11-72.

von der Heide, S., G. Emons, R. Hilgers, and V. Viereck. "Effect on Muscles of Mechanical Vibrations Produced by the Galileo 2000 in Combination with Physical Therapy in Treating Female Stress Urinary Incontinence."

Harmful Consequences

Kleinöder, H., J. Ziegler, C. Bosse, and J. Mester. "Safety Considerations in Vibration Training." Institute of Training and Movement Science, German Sport University Cologne.

Resources and Additional Reading

Resources

Becky Chambers, Naturopath, BS, MEd
Vibrant Health
www.BCVibrantHealth.com

Candida Yeast

Chaitow, Leon. *Candida Albicans: Could Yeast Be Your Problem?* Rochester, VT: Healing Arts Press, 1998.

Crook, William. *The Yeast Connection: A Medical Breakthrough.* Berkeley, CA: Crown Publishing Group, 1994

Trowbridge, John Parks, and Morton Walker. *The Yeast Syndrome.* New York: Bantam Books, 1985.

Wunderlich, Ray Jr., and Dwight Kalita. *The Candida Yeast Syndrome.* New York: McGraw-Hill, 1998.

Physical Therapy

Albasini, Alfio, Martin Krause, and Ingo Volker Rembitzki. *Using Whole Body Vibration in Physical Therapy and Sport: Clinical Practice and Treatment Exercises*. Edinburgh; New York: Churchill Livingstone/Elsevier, 2010.

Toxins and Detoxification

Rogers, Sherry A. *Detoxify or Die*. Sarasota, FL: Sand Key Company, 2002. http://prestigepublishing.com/cgi-bin/start.cgi/apps/cartcompanion/category.html

About the Author

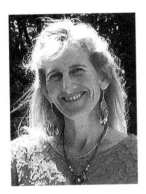 Becky Chambers is a naturopath, teacher, author, and the president and owner of Vibrant Health, where she specializes in the breakthrough body, mind, and energy therapy of Whole Body Vibration. As the first and most experienced expert in Whole Body Vibration in the Northeast, Becky is the area's foremost provider of this revolutionary technology. Becky has a bachelor of science degree in biology from the University of Massachusetts, a master's in education from Lesley College, and she graduated with highest honors from Clayton College of Natural Health with a Doctor of Naturopathy degree in 2003.

She has spent the last twenty years discovering powerful new energy therapies that have led to a transformation of her life on every level. She has also published a memoir, *Beyond the Great Abyss: A True Story of Transformation through Natural Health Breakthroughs*.

Please visit her website at www.BCVibrantHealth.com.